I AM
BEAUTY

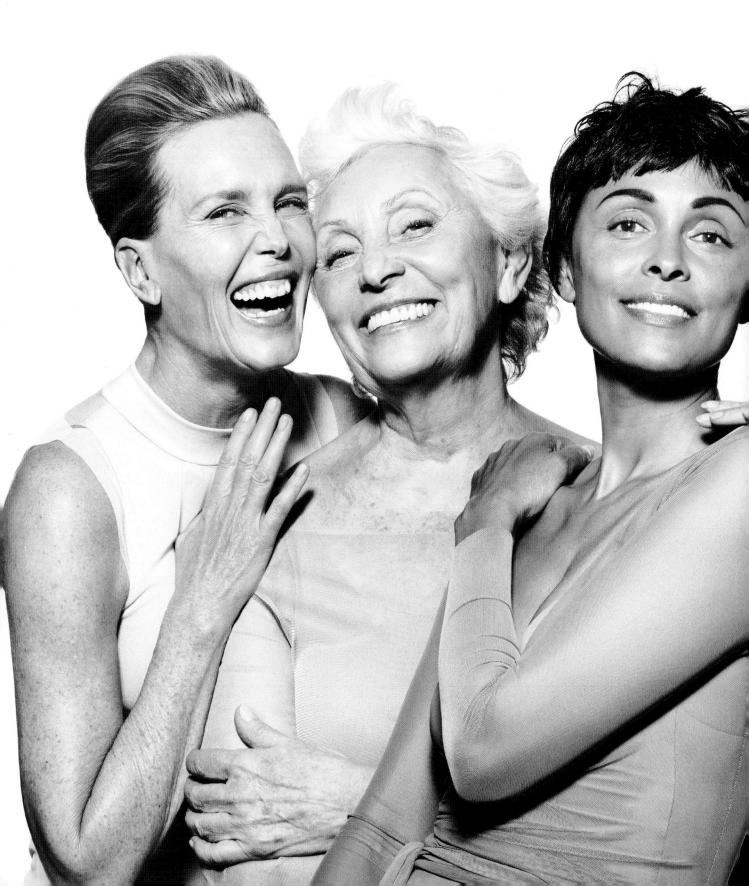

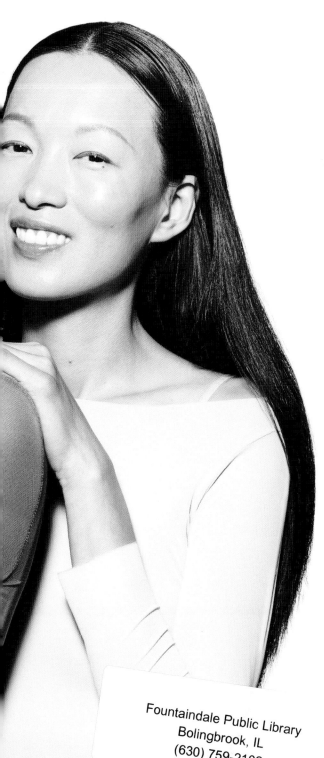

I AM BEAUTY

Timeless Skincare and Beauty
for Women 40 and Over

RIKU CAMPO

Photography by Samantha Rapp

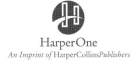

HarperOne
An Imprint of HarperCollinsPublishers

HarperOne

Photography by Samantha Rapp

The beauty advice presented in this book is intended only as an informative resource guide to help you make informed decisions; it is not meant to replace the advice of a physician or to serve as a guide to self-treatment. Always seek competent medical help for any health condition or if there is any question about the appropriateness of a procedure or recommendation.

HarperCollins books may be purchased for educational, business, or sales promotional use. For information, please email the Special Markets Department at SPsales@harpercollins.com.

FIRST EDITION

Library of Congress Cataloging-in-Publication Data

Names: Campo, Riku, author.
Title: I am beauty: timeless skincare and beauty for women 40 and over / Riku Campo.

Description: First edition. | San Francisco: HarperOne, 2020

Identifiers: LCCN 2019033517 (print) | LCCN 2019033518 (ebook) |
ISBN 9780062946454 (hardcover) | ISBN 9780062946447 (ebook)

Subjects: LCSH: Beauty, Personal. | Middle-aged women—Care and hygiene. | Cosmetics

Classification: LCC RA776.98 .C36 2020 (print) | LCC RA776.98 (ebook) |
DDC 646.7/20844—dc23

LC record available at https://lccn.loc.gov/2019033517
LC ebook record available at https://lccn.loc.gov/2019033518

20 21 22 23 24   TC   10 9 8 7 6 5 4 3 2 1

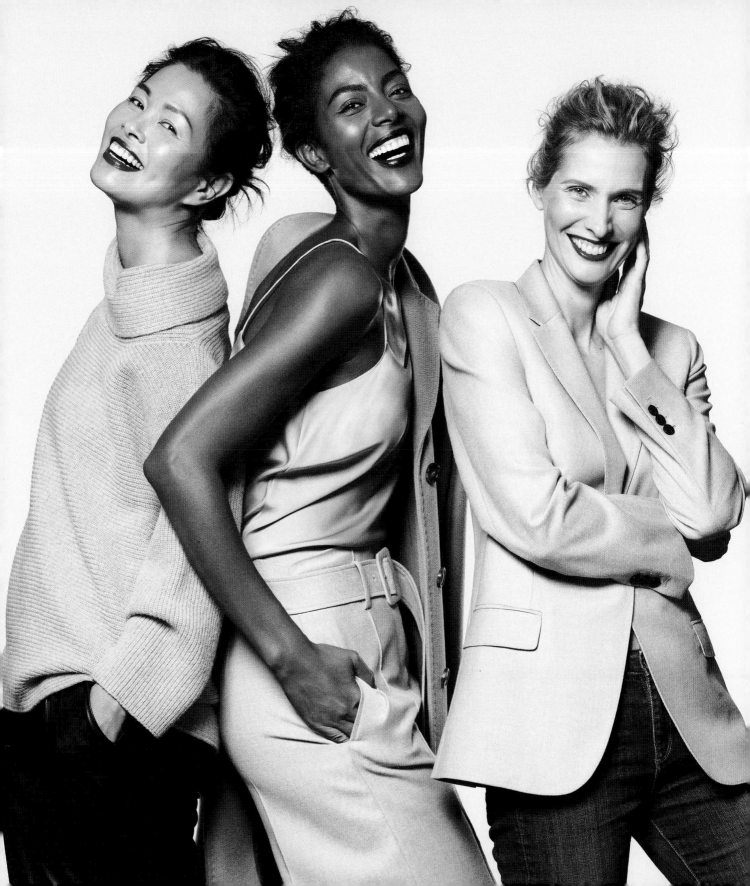

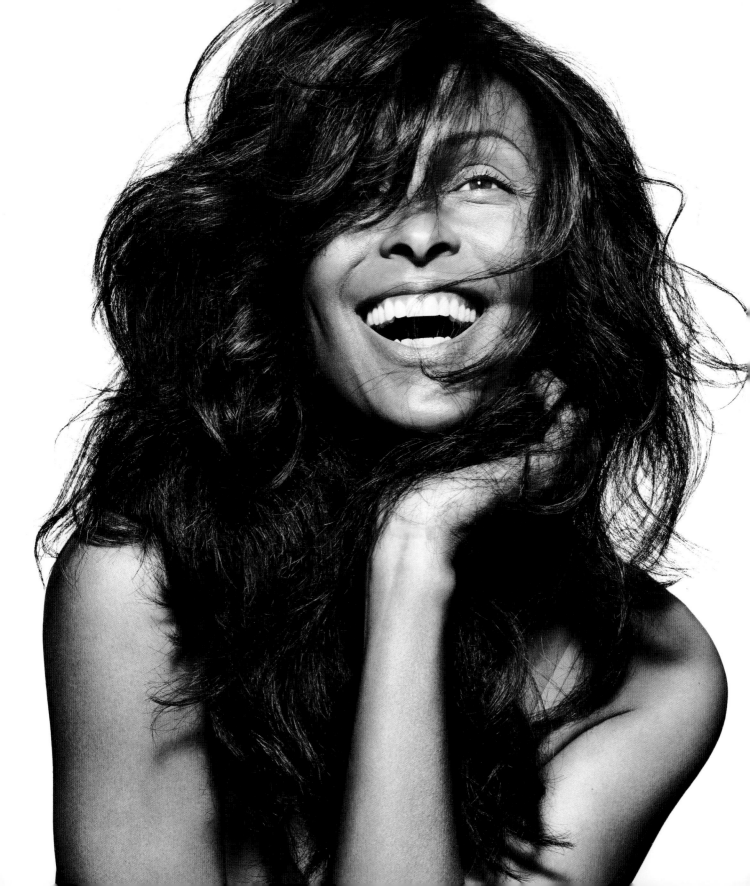

Hello!

My name is Riku.

This book is dedicated to my mother, Inkeri, who taught me how important it is to be kind to one another and that kindness channels beauty—the inner beauty that shows on your face through confidence and smiling eyes.

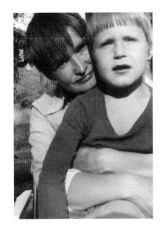

I started out wanting to create a book for mature women whose beauty is enhanced by age. But I also wanted to create a book that would portray women over 40 in a new light and update old-fashioned stereotypes.

So this book is also dedicated to all women over 40—mothers and daughters, every race and size, every sexual orientation and gender identity, and every nationality. Be visible, get inspired, and find new ideas for your everyday beauty routines. I was lucky to have photographer Samantha Rapp on my team, because she understood my vision and created images that highlight every model's individual beauty.

Be curious, enjoy life, enjoy yourself, and enjoy this book. Let's celebrate you!

Cheers for life,
Riku

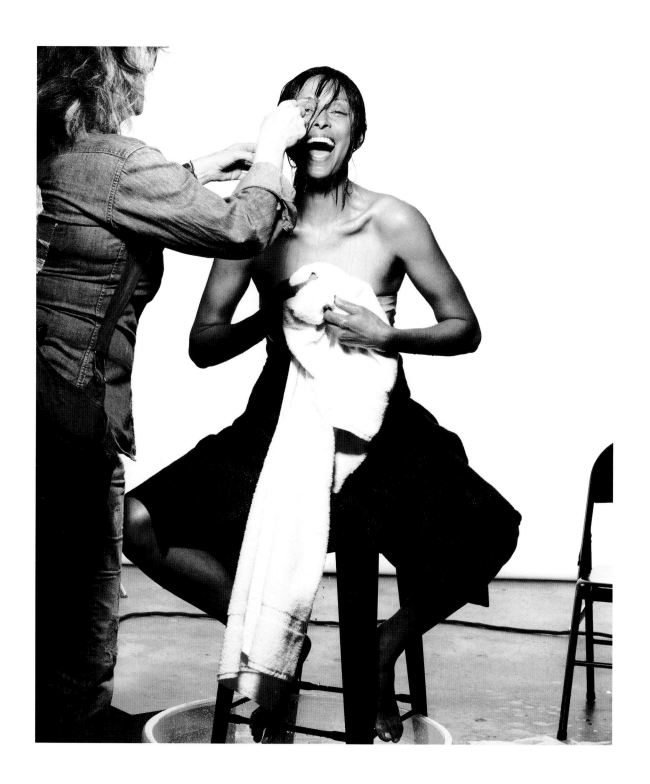

Photographer's Note

Now that I am in my 40s, I have embraced the changes in my skincare routine and my relationship to makeup that growing older brings. When I was in my 20s, a light moisturizer and lip balm did the trick. I was out the door without giving a thought to sunscreen, night cream, or eye cream. Much has changed.

At an age when your list of required makeup and skincare products typically increases, you notice that there isn't much representation of older women in the beauty market. This project set out to expand the conversation and celebrate women of every age.

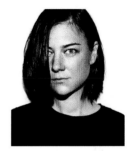

It was an absolute privilege to work with these amazing women— each brought a unique joy and energy to the shoots, and we worked in a truly collaborative fashion. We chose to start each sitting with a "naked" face portrait. Very quickly I realized that regardless of their varying levels of experience in front of a camera, all the women who came through the studio had an inner radiance that was infectious and undeniable. Their beaming expressions set the tone for the day.

Traditionally, beauty images are shot from very close up, concentrating only on the face and the makeup. We thought it was important to pull the camera back so we could show finished looks and highlight the styling and accessorizing for each, an approach unique to this book. This, we felt, would help the reader select a makeup look suitable for her personal style. After all, we usually coordinate our makeup choices with what we have in the closet, whether we're going to work, getting ready for an evening out, or preparing to go on vacation.

Have some fun, take some chances, experiment with color or a new technique. Grab a few new brushes, add to your collection of tried-and-true lip colors, and express yourself.

We should all celebrate our uniqueness, our voices, and our ages—whether 20 or 85. Own it!

Samantha Rapp

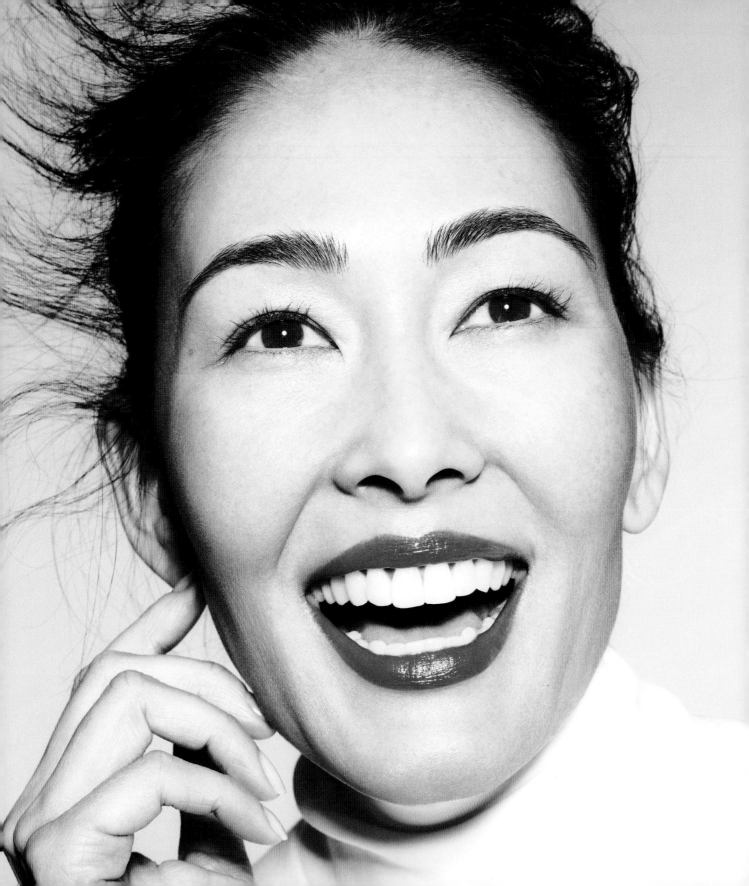

CONTENTS

PART I: FUNDAMENTALS OF BEAUTY

PART II: BEAUTY IN ACTION

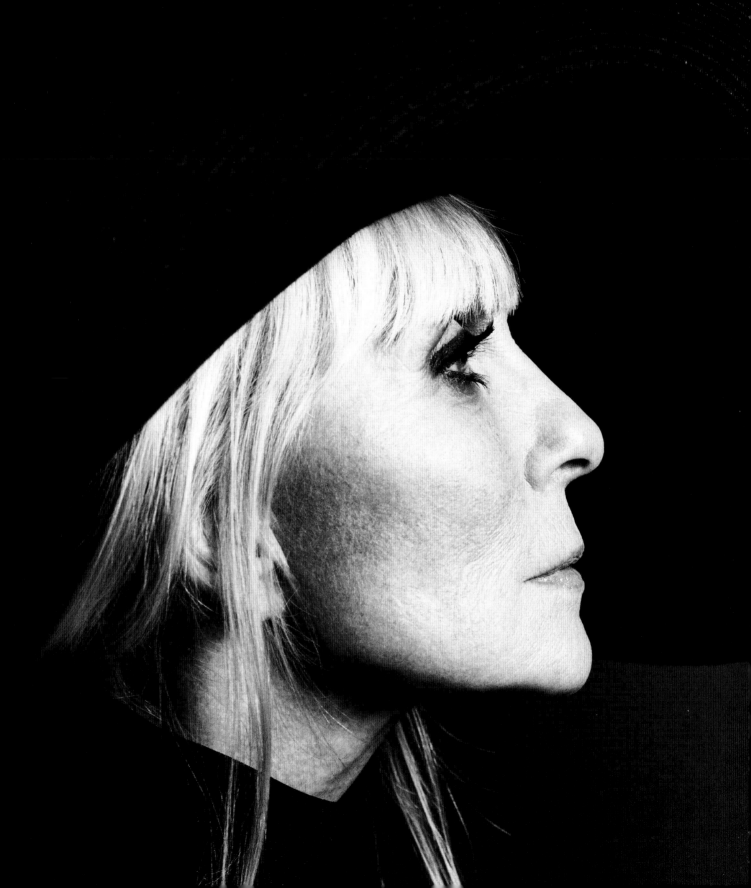

I

FUNDAMENTALS
of BEAUTY

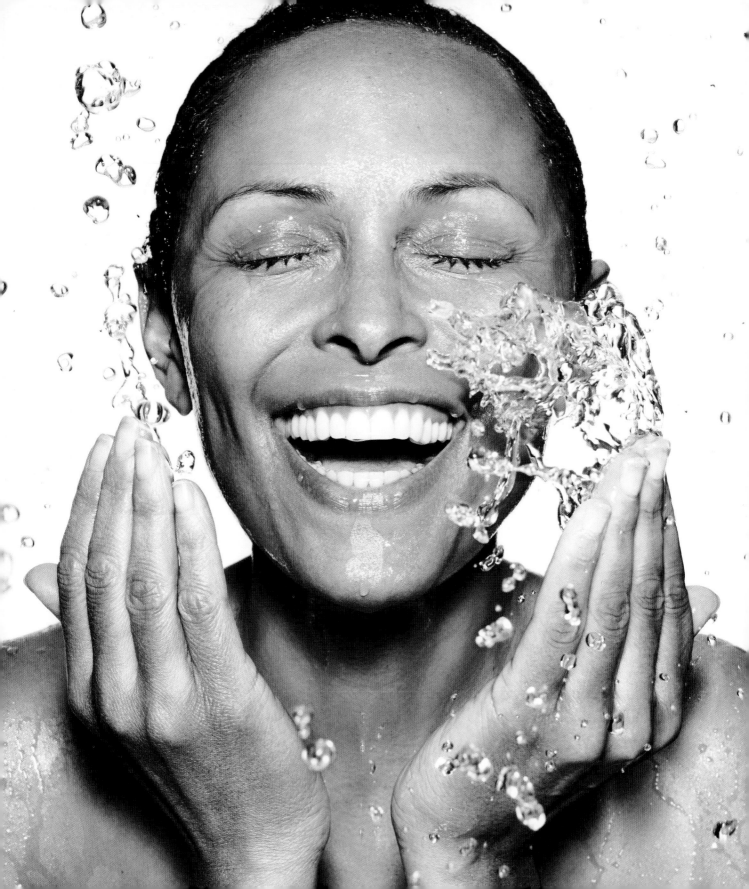

1

SKINCARE

We all know the importance of a daily skincare routine, and in my opinion this vital process shouldn't take more than a few minutes in the morning and evening.

Following are the products I recommend for optimal skincare:

- Cleansing milk (shelf life: one year)—use during cold months

- Cleansing foam (shelf life: one year)—washes sunscreen off better and faster than other cleansers, according to New York City dermatologist Dr. Ellen Marmur

- Toner (shelf life: six months)

- Eye cream (shelf life: one year)

- Serum (shelf life: one year)—skincare product used after the toner on clean skin and before moisturizer and sunscreen

- Day cream and night cream (shelf life: eighteen months)—always wash your hands before using creams, or use a spatula to scrape the cream from the jar

- Sunscreen (shelf life: two years)—be sure to choose one with a minimum SPF of 30 as well as UVA and UVB protection

- Lip balm (shelf life: one to two years)

- Exfoliant (shelf life: one year)—use any exfoliation or face scrub product

- Face mask (shelf life: one year)

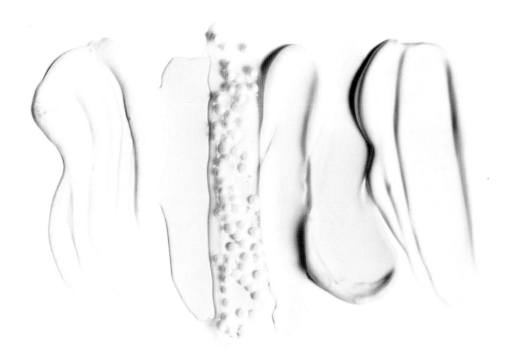

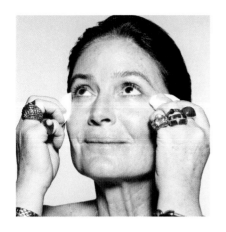
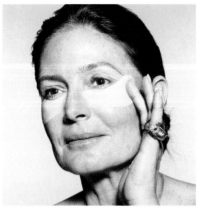
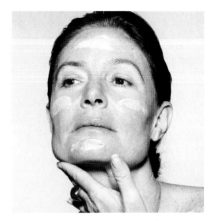

MORNING ROUTINE

Wash your face

Because skin gets drier with age, you might need a product designed for dry and sensitive skin, such as cleansing milk. If you have combination or oily skin, however, choose a cleansing foam.

Apply toner

Toner cleanses and closes the pores as well as corrects and balances the pH of your skin. I like spray toners—they are like a cool mini shower for your face! Gel toners are also an excellent choice.

Moisturize the eye area

The skin around your eyes is the thinnest on your body and loses moisture quickly, so an eye cream is essential for your daily skincare routine, morning and night. If you have particularly dry skin or puffy eyes in the morning, get under-eye patches or eye pens. These smooth the skin, reduce puffiness, and fight dark circles.

Apply serum

Buy a serum that contains skin-firming ingredients such as vitamin C, hyaluronic acid, or retinol (vitamin A). Retinol makes your skin more sensitive to the sun, so don't forget to add SPF-60 sunscreen on top of the serum and moisturizer. On a warm summer day, you can skip the moisturizer and add your sunscreen on top of your serum.

Apply day cream

Most people over 40 have dry skin, so I recommend using a thick face cream, especially during fall and winter, to ultramoisturize your skin. Don't forget to moisturize your neck as well.

Apply sunscreen

Dermatologists recommend applying sunscreen with an SPF of 60 all over your face, ears, neck, and hands. You can apply your makeup directly on top of this.

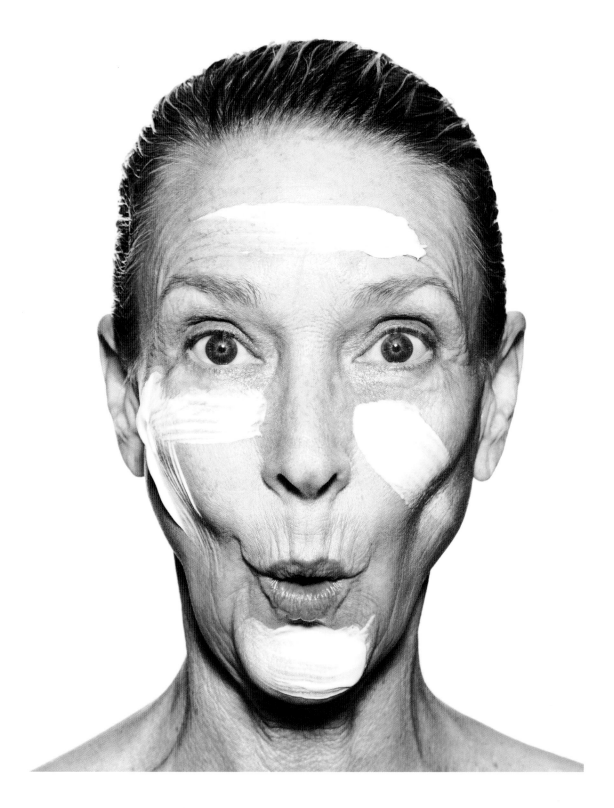

EVENING ROUTINE AND EXTRA CARE

Wash your face

Cleanse twice at night.

Apply toner, eye cream, and serum

Repeat your morning routine with these three steps.

Apply night cream

At night your cells are most active, so your skin naturally repairs itself while you sleep. Massage the night cream into your face—this relaxes your face muscles and allows the cream to absorb faster.

Exfoliate

This removes the dead skin cells on your face, neck, and chest. You can use a mild exfoliant three times a week.

Use a face mask

If your skin is dry, choose a cream mask that you can leave on your skin overnight. Face-mask sheets are also very handy. After you peel off the mask, let your skin sit and absorb the ingredients. You can massage your face at the same time and spread the product on your neck. Use it three times a week.

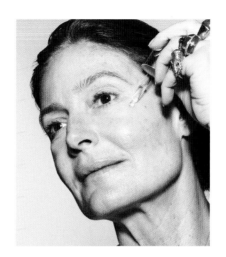
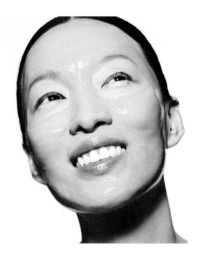
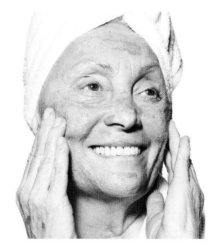

SOS SKINCARE

Do you have a pimple in the middle of your forehead? Do you have dry, flaky skin or puffy eyes after a long night of celebration? If you need to get back to normal as soon as possible, follow these tips for immediate results.

Super-dry skin

In the winter or after a long airline flight, it's time to get some extra help. Drink lots of water to hydrate your skin from the inside out. Exfoliate your face and neck, and apply a facial oil all over your skin. Let it absorb for a few minutes before applying a thick moisturizer. This can work as a face mask if you apply more cream than normal, covering your face completely with moisturizer. Leave it for fifteen to twenty minutes, and afterward, press tissues firmly on your skin to take off the extra cream.

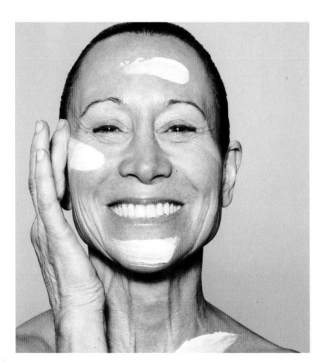

Pimples

Instead of popping blemishes, apply an acne spot-treatment gel that contains maximum-strength salicylic acid. This will penetrate pores, shrink blemishes, and clear the skin. Let it dry for five minutes, then apply an acne patch and leave it on overnight. For an organic treatment, try tea tree oil, a strong antiseptic and anti-inflammatory home remedy. Azulene, derived from chamomile, also works for these purposes, says aesthetician Gaby Niessen at Verabella Spa in Beverly Hills. As you put on your makeup, apply concealer to the pimple with a small brush. Add a small amount of transparent powder on top to finish.

Puffy eyes

Using ice cubes to relieve puffy eyes is an old Hollywood beauty trick. Gently glide the cube across the under-eye area, back and forth. When it starts to feel too cold, set the ice cube down and tap your index and middle fingers around the whole eye area for around one minute. Repeat these steps three times. This will help boost circulation and detoxify the lymphatic system. Then tap the eye area dry and apply under-eye patches for fifteen minutes. After that, tap on the eye area for one more minute, and the puffiness should be settled.

You can also use cooled, steeped green-tea bags instead of eye patches. Green tea contains the anti-inflammatory ingredient EGCG (epigallocatechin gallate), along with antioxidants, tannins, and caffeine, which will constrict blood vessels. Let the tea bags chill and leave them under the eyes for ten to fifteen minutes while you're lying down.

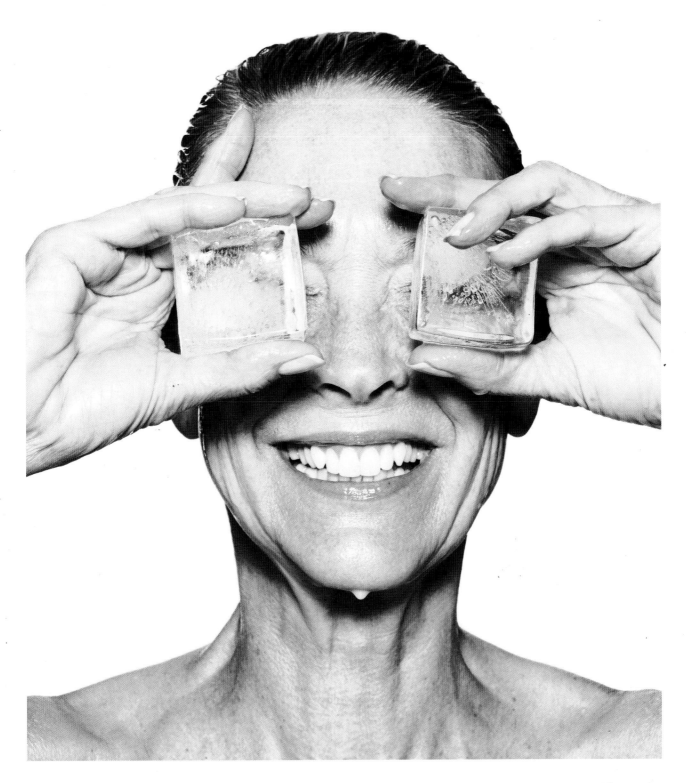

Cracked lips

Most often, a simple lip balm can heal cracked lips. However, licking your lips too much, sunburn, and allergies can exacerbate dry lips. Niessen suggests opening a vitamin E capsule with a needle and applying the liquid straight to your lips. This promotes cell turnover and moisturization.

Pillow marks

Glide ice cubes across the skin gently—this will make the pillow marks disappear faster. To avoid pillow marks, use silk pillowcases.

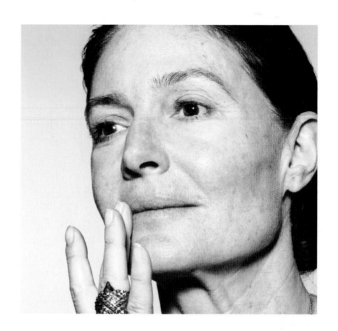

MOST POWERFUL SKINCARE INGREDIENTS

Hyaluronic acid

This replenishes moisture in dry skin.

Vitamin C

This antioxidant combats free radicals, brightens your skin tone, and reduces sun damage and age spots.

Retinol (vitamin A)

This most powerful antiaging ingredient stimulates collagen production, tightens pores, and evens out skin tone.

Vitamin E

This antioxidant brightens and moisturizes your skin and reduces inflammation.

Peptides

These increase collagen production and therefore reduce wrinkles.

Green tea

This powerful antioxidant combats free radicals and rejuvenates your skin.

Stem cells

These increase production of collagen and repair damaged cells.

Ceramides

The body produces these natural lipids to help your skin maintain its moisture level.

Glycolic acid

This exfoliant removes dead skin cells, smooths the skin, and reduces fine lines.

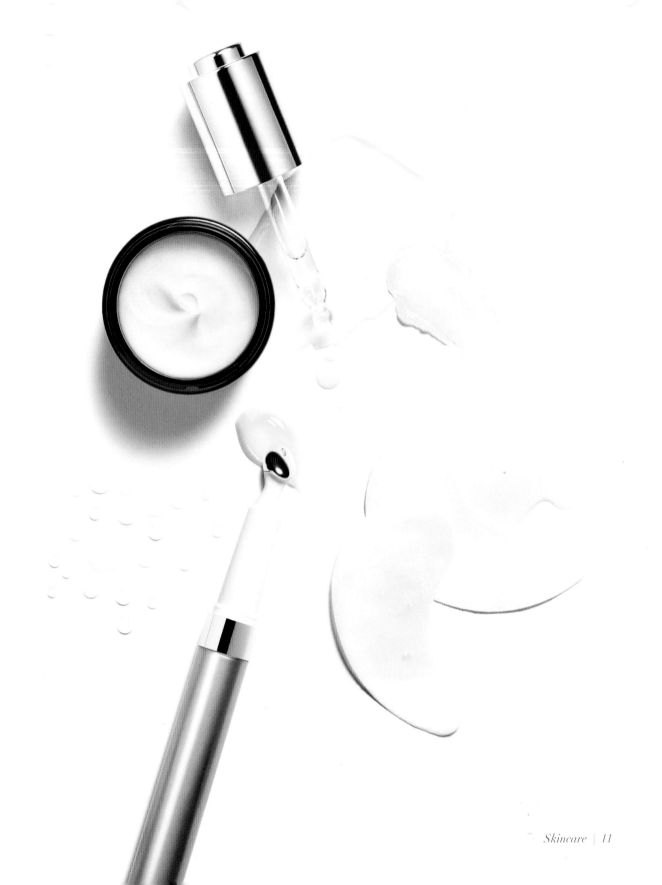

PRE-MAKEUP FACIAL

I have worked as a makeup artist for more than thirty years, and skincare has always been my first love—my passion. I start every client's makeup application with a mini facial, and you can easily replicate this at home.

1. Cleanse the face with cleansing milk.

2. Apply toner with cotton pads. This will clean the pores of dirt, sunscreen, and any remaining makeup.

3. Apply a moisturizing face-mask sheet and leave it on for around 10 minutes.

4. Apply a rich moisturizer (unless your skin is oily—in that case, use oil-free moisturizer) and massage it into the skin.

5. Massage your skin by tapping on it with your fingers—like playing piano on your face—for five minutes. This works especially well in the morning if your skin looks tired and puffy.

6. If you're going to be outdoors, apply an SPF-60 sunscreen with UVA and UVB protection.

After this small facial routine, the skin looks much more alive and takes on a special glow.

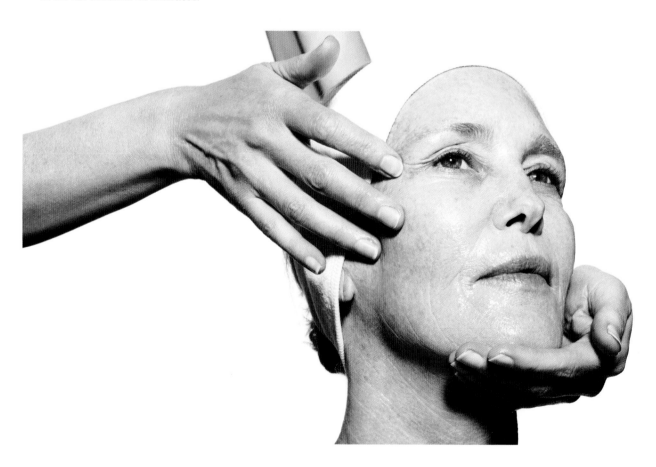

HOW TO GIVE YOURSELF A FACIAL MASSAGE

Facial massages are very important for women over 40 because they increase blood circulation and oxygen flow to the muscles in the face. They also stimulate the fascia (the connective tissue between your skin and facial muscles), which can help smooth out and prevent fine lines—an instant face-lift. My basic technique, below, will also relax the face muscles and relieve tension.

1. Make sure your face and hands are clean and your hair is pulled off your face.

2. Apply face oil or moisturizing cream on your skin and neck.

3. Massage these seven areas:

    a. Lower neck up to the chin

    b. Lower jaw toward the ears

    c. Chin toward the ears

    d. Outer corner of the lips toward the ears

    e. Outer corner of the nose to the temple

    f. Around the nose

    g. The forehead (with an upward motion)

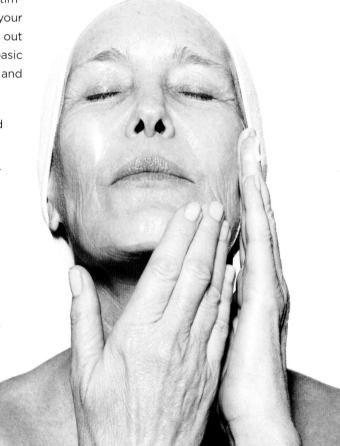

ADVICE FROM AESTHETICIANS AND DERMATOLOGISTS

I've always been interested in skincare because I grew up with genetic atopic eczema, and I was recently diagnosed with rosacea. When I was a young boy in Finland, I remember waking up for school an hour early to moisturize my skin from head to toe so I wouldn't develop dry areas and rashes on my face and neck. The long, extremely cold winters didn't help, either.

Thankfully, in the course of my work, I have met some of the best aestheticians and dermatologists in the world, and they've helped me keep my skin as healthy as it can possibly be. Below, they share their advice for skin of all types.

If you have adult acne, rosacea, psoriasis, or eczema, I highly recommend you consult a specialist for a personalized treatment plan.

Nachi

Aesthetician at Mist Beauty by Nachi, New York City

How often do you recommend having a facial?

Usually I advise my clients to have a facial every four to six weeks. However, it really depends on your skin type. Some of my clients are absolutely fine waiting two to three months between facials.

Is there a difference between a facial for a woman in her 20s and a facial for a woman over 40?

Women in their late 40s and over have very different skin concerns from those of women in their 20s. Once you are in your 40s, you have less elastin and collagen, and you tend to produce less oil and water, resulting in dry skin. Facials for women in this age range need to address these issues.

What are the benefits of facials?

Deep cleansing of your skin—including the removal of blackheads, whiteheads, and milia—as well as exfoliation results in brighter, healthier, and more toned skin. It also improves absorption and thus the efficacy of skincare products. In addition, facials are very good at targeting specific problems such as acne scars, pigmentation issues, fine lines, and dry skin. There isn't necessarily any magic to this, but skincare products tend to be more effective when applied by a professional. The best analogy I can think of is the difference between brushing your teeth and getting your teeth cleaned by a dental hygienist. The home treatment is important, but the professional is able to focus on specific areas, yielding even better results.

Skin becomes drier as we age. What can we do to make it more hydrated?

I firmly believe that diet and nutrition have an enormous effect on the skin. If you want to keep your skin hydrated, drink at least two liters of water per day and eat a lot of vegetables and collagen-rich foods (for example, wild salmon, citrus fruits, berries, pumpkin seeds, eggs, and avocados). I also recommend incorporating a skin supplement such as hyaluronic acid or collagen into your daily routine.

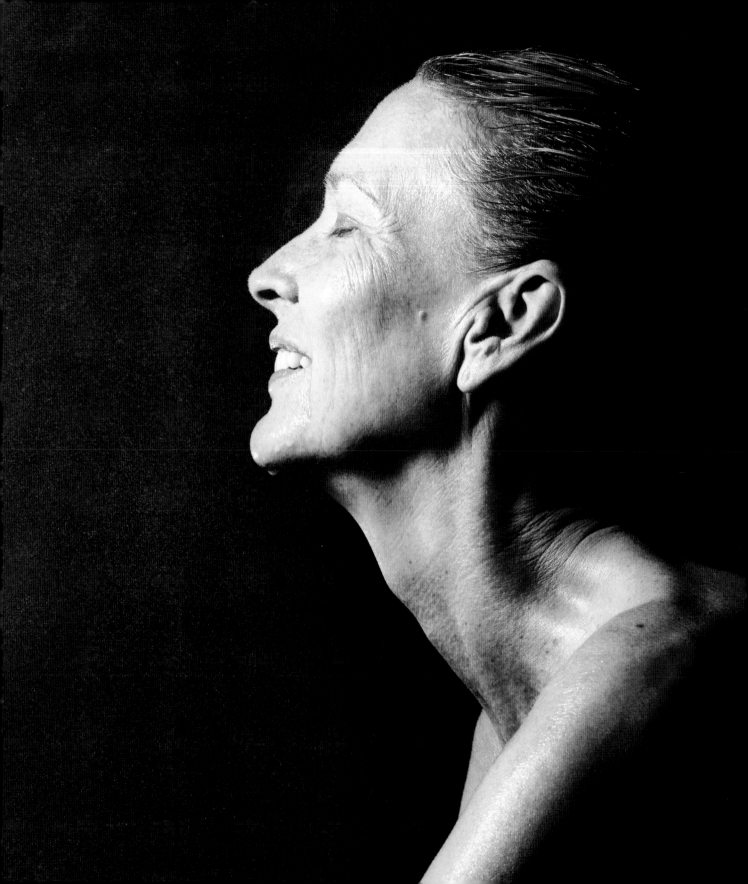

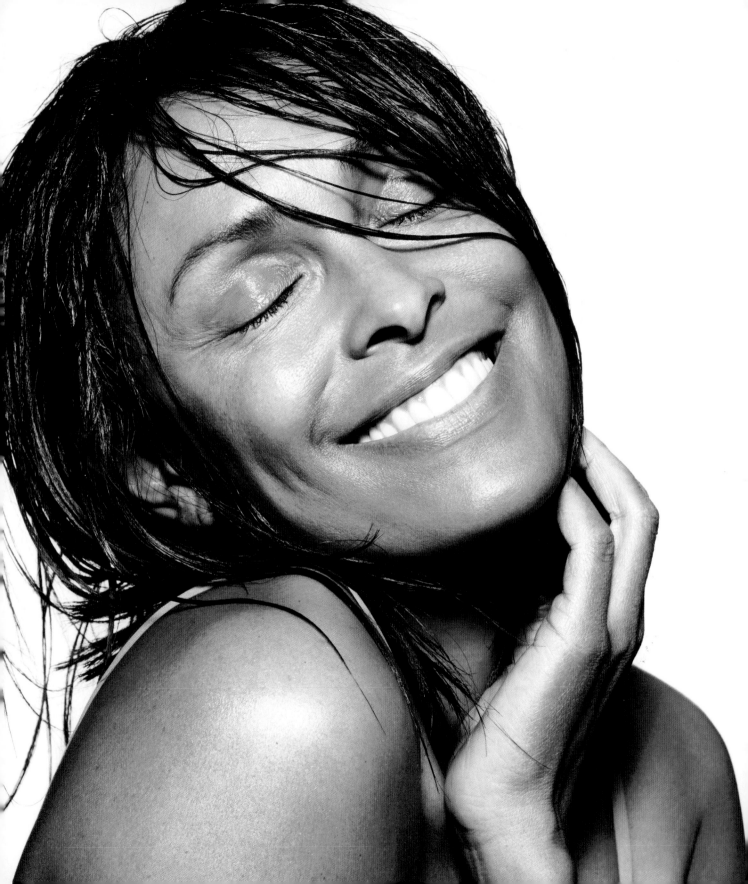

Danielle Gamble

Lead Aesthetician at Sisley Paris, New York City

What are the main reasons you recommend facials to women (and men) over 40?

Unfortunately, collagen production declines as we age. We can benefit from the stimulation that comes from facials. A regular facial massage can help prevent dull skin and help achieve that youthful glow we all admire. Facials also help relax tight muscles in the face, which often are responsible for wrinkles. Lymphatic drainage, a favorite massage technique of mine, is especially helpful in reducing puffiness. Facials are the ultimate antiaging weapon.

What are the most important steps for skincare at home?

Double-cleanse every single night. Repair at night with serums and moisturizers. Protect during the day. Those tips are nonnegotiable.

What is the correct way to apply product to the eye area?

Use your ring finger, because it allows for gentle application. Starting at the inner corner, gently tap or glide your finger around the orbital bone. No pulling.

What are milia, and how do you get rid of them?

Milia form because of a buildup of keratin in the outermost layer of the skin. These painless bumps are very common, especially around the eyes, and some people are more prone to them than others. They can go away on their own, but often you need an aesthetician or a doctor to remove them. Using a lancet, a professional will poke a tiny hole and push the milium out. The hole should be so tiny that no mark will be left. Do not try squeezing it on your own. That will leave a mark.

Michele S. Green, MD

Cosmetic Dermatologist, New York City

How does the skin change between the ages of 40 and 55?

During those years, wrinkles are more prominent, because the skin loses its elasticity. The skin around the eyelids starts drooping, and the lines are deeper along the forehead and glabella (the skin between the eyebrows and above the nose). Hyperpigmentation (dark spots and sun spots) may appear or become more visible as a result of years of UV exposure. These spots may appear on the hands, chest, and neck in addition to the face. Because of the loss of elasticity and reduced collagen production, slackness becomes more severe, especially in the lower face (the jowls, the corners of the mouth) and the neck.

How about between the ages of 55 and 65?

As we go into our mid-50s, estrogen levels drop, which, along with environmental damage, can contribute to premature aging. Also, the epidermis thins, cell turnover slows down, and there is a substantial loss of function. In aging skin we need to both reverse the damage and prevent further deterioration. Ultraviolet light causes thousands of cellular DNA alterations each day, resulting in cumulative damage to the skin. Environmental pollutants such as cigarette smoke also accelerate the natural aging process.

In addition, as skin ages, keratinocytes change shape and become shorter while corneocytes become bigger as a result of decreased epidermal turnover. [Keratinocytes are found in the outermost layer of the skin, the epidermis. Corneocytes are terminally differentiated keratinocytes and compose all the outermost part of the epidermis.] Sebum decreases significantly—as much as 60 percent—and enzymatically active melanocytes [melanin-producing cells] decrease at a rate of 8 to 20 percent per decade, resulting in uneven pigmentation. There is also loss of natural water in the skin, and the lipid content decreases. With this lower water content, skin undergoes a significant reduction in its barrier function and appears drier. In addition, we see a decrease in collagen turnover as well as elastin production. The overall volume of subcutaneous fat decreases until around age seventy, which gives individuals of that age a hollow look.

And then between the ages of 65 and 75?

The skin loses fat in the subcutaneous layers, which causes the appearance of sagging skin around the temples, eyes, cheeks, and chin.

What can women over 50 do to keep their skin healthy?

Aging skin needs facials that are hydrating and firming, so women over 50 should have those types of facials once a month. In addition, they should undergo other beauty treatments that will stimulate collagen production, such as Thermage radiofrequency treatments and vampire facials (microneedling followed by the application of PRP, or platelet-rich plasma). Oxygen facials are a great way to boost radiance and

skin health because they increase the absorption of topical vitamins and minerals.

What kind of diet and lifestyle changes are best for optimal skin health?

It's important to add more vegetables and fruits to your daily diet. Consume foods that contain healthful oils and fats as well as those high in vitamins and calcium. Drink alcohol in moderation because alcohol can also worsen age-related health conditions, including high blood pressure, diabetes, and memory problems. Increase your bone density by engaging in strength training and weight-bearing exercise and taking collagen supplements. It is also very important to increase your protein intake, because 50 percent of your bones are made of protein. You should also maintain a diet high in calcium, the most important mineral for bone health. Vitamins D and K help your body absorb calcium.

[Vitamins play a huge role in skin health, particularly vitamin A/retinoid. Beef, eggs, and dairy are good sources of vitamin A. Vitamin B3/niacin is great for aged skin because it brightens the skin's appearance and reduces redness; all animal and plant foods are good sources. Vitamin B5 prevents water loss from the skin and improves skin barrier functioning; it can be found in whole grains, avocado, and chicken. Vitamin C creates collagen, which keeps your skin firm and protects your skin from free-radical damage; sources include tomatoes, lemons, grapefruit, strawberries, and broccoli. Vitamin D defends your skin against acne and other infections; milk, fish, and eggs provide ample amounts, and if you don't live in a sunny area, you should take supplements. Vitamin E protects

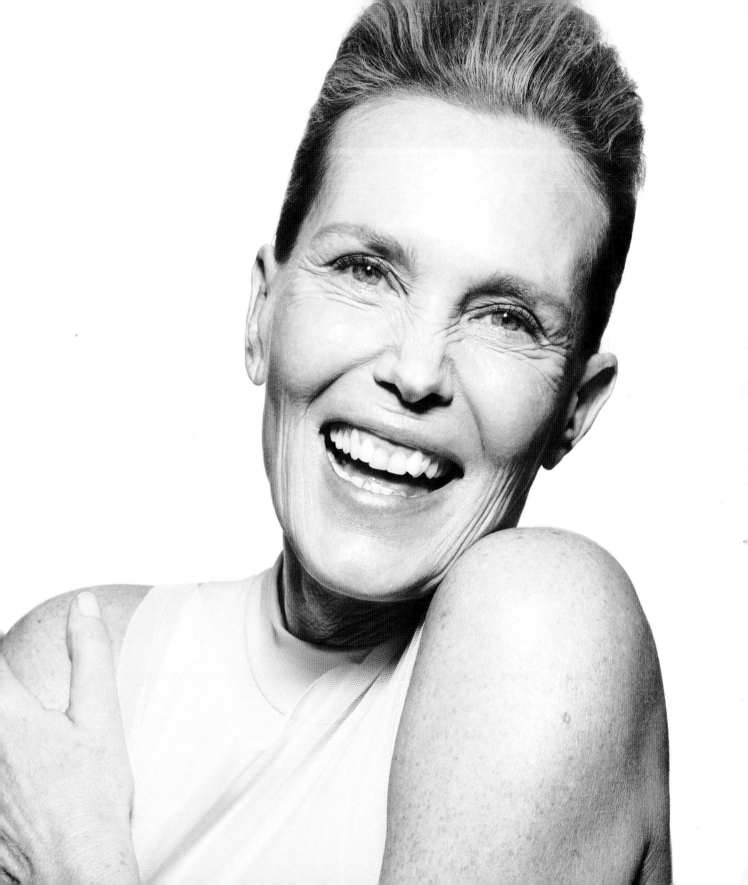

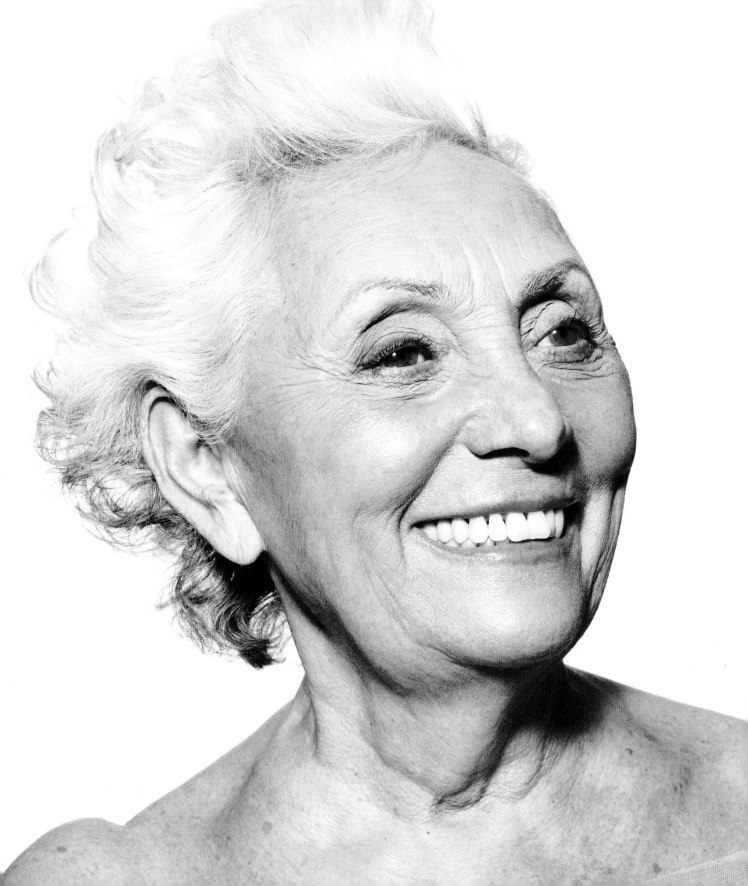

your skin from free-radical damage and is found in vegetables, fruits, nuts, and seeds. Vitamin K heals wounds and bruises; cabbage, liver, kale, and milk supply it.]

What is the best sunscreen for the face and body? For example, what is the difference between SPF 40 and SPF 80?

Choose a broad-spectrum sunscreen that has both UVA and UVB protection. An SPF of 30 or more is recommended. However, if you have a history of skin cancer, suffer from melasma (a skin condition in which brown patches appear on the face) or hyperpigmentation, or tend to burn quickly, you should consider an SPF of 60 or more. The SPF number tells you how long it takes for the sun to affect your skin. For example, an SPF of 40 means it takes forty minutes of sun exposure before your skin starts getting red. In addition, SPF 40 and SPF 30 allow 3 percent of the sun's UV rays to penetrate the skin, while SPF 80 and SPF 60 allow only 2 percent.

Does sunscreen work as an antiaging product?

The sun is the number one cause of wrinkles; dozens of studies have documented its impact. Avoiding sun exposure during peak hours (10:00 a.m. to 4:00 p.m.) can reduce sun damage by as much 60 percent. If you can't avoid outdoor activities during these peak times, wear protective clothing, a hat, and sunglasses. Reapply sunscreen every two hours. Wearing sunscreen every single day can slow or even prevent the development of wrinkles and sagging skin. Just remember to apply sunscreen every time you go outside and that it takes fifteen minutes to absorb.

What is the best way to remove brown spots?

Laser treatment is the most effective. The Alex TriVantage dual-wavelength laser can be used to treat dark spots and deep lesions effectively. There is little or no downtime with this laser.

If a woman wants to tighten her skin a little, what nonsurgical treatments are available?

The Fraxel laser treatment—a type of fractional resurfacing—penetrates the superficial layers of the skin, treating fine lines and wrinkles and improving overall tone and texture. The results of Fraxel treatment can be seen immediately; however, the full effects are seen after four weeks. It works with the body's natural healing process to produce smoother, brighter skin with minimal downtime. It also removes sun damage, brown spots, and fine lines.

As I mentioned earlier, Thermage is a noninvasive procedure that uses radiofrequency technology and is effective for all skin types. It releases heat energy beneath the dermis, regenerating collagen and resulting in smoother, tighter skin.

Aquagold, a type of microneedling treatment, uses twenty-four-karat-gold needles, each of which is thinner than a strand of hair. It allows the ingredients (a mixture of Botox, Restylane, and antioxidants) to penetrate six hundred microns deep, rejuvenating and lightening the skin.

PRP used in microneedling treatments, stimulates cell turnover and collagen production by creating tiny microchannels in the skin. As the skin heals, the cells stimulate collagen production. The result is younger-looking skin.

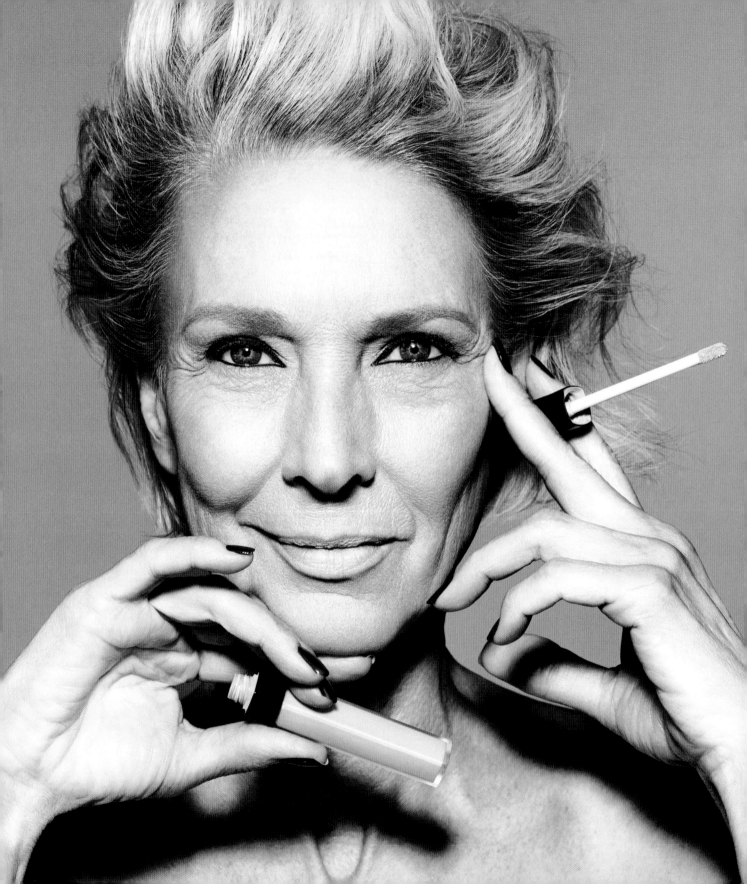

BUYING and USING COSMETICS

I want your makeup to be so simple that you can easily do it yourself. The secret is good-quality makeup. You don't need to use five different eye shadows, mix three lipstick colors, or contour and highlight endlessly to create a look that is far from who you are. For me, makeup is not art on your face but rather an expression of your identity. So ladies, let's keep the makeup real, simple, and easy!

When you're shopping for makeup, I always recommend stepping into the store, taking your time, looking around, asking questions, and letting a makeup artist or sales professional try it on your face. That's why they're there. If you don't try it, you might end up buying a product that doesn't work for your skin type, doesn't match your complexion, has a weird texture, or doesn't suit your skin tone. And remember that even if your best friend recommends her all-time favorite lipstick color or foundation, it might not work for you.

Most important, take what is helpful for you and leave the rest. Depending on your daily routine and style, you may not need a lot of cosmetics—the list below is only meant to inspire you. Maybe you just want a touch of concealer, mascara, and lip stain. Or maybe you want the full makeup experience every day—and that's perfectly okay! That's part of what makes you *you*.

These are the products I find essential:

- Tinted moisturizer or a lightweight hydrating foundation (shelf life: one year)—we'll discuss how to find the right one for your skin in chapter 3

- Concealer and/or color corrector (shelf life: eighteen months)

- Loose powder (shelf life: one to three years, depending upon how clean you keep your brush)

- Eyebrow pencil or eyebrow powder compact (shelf life: two years)

- Mascara (shelf life: three months)

- Matte eye shadow (shelf life: two to three years if you keep your brushes clean)

- Eye pencil or liquid liner (shelf life: two years for pencils, one year for liquids)

CARE AND KEEPING OF MAKEUP BRUSHES

When you use good-quality brushes, makeup application is smooth and fast, and when you take good care of your brushes, they can last decades. I have some brushes I bought in Paris in 1990, and I use them daily.

- Using warm soapy water, wash your foundation and concealer brushes one to two times a week. Wash the rest of your brushes every other week.

- After washing the brushes, let them air-dry on a towel.

- You can also quick-wash brushes that you don't use for foundation or concealer by using a brush-cleaner spray.

- At home, keep your brushes in a drinking glass so they don't lie on the bathroom counter. This also makes it easier to find the brush you need.

- Get a small brush case that you can keep in your purse for touch-ups. It's more hygienic than letting the brushes bounce around freely in your makeup bag.

- Lipstick, lip gloss, and lip pencil (shelf life: two years for lipsticks, one year for lip glosses, and two years for pencils)

- Blush or bronzer (shelf life: 1 year for creams, a few years for powders)

Keep your skincare and makeup products in a bathroom cabinet, away from heat and sunlight.

Below is a list of the twelve makeup brushes I used on the sixteen women featured in this book. You don't need all these brushes, but I want to show you what they are and what they can do.

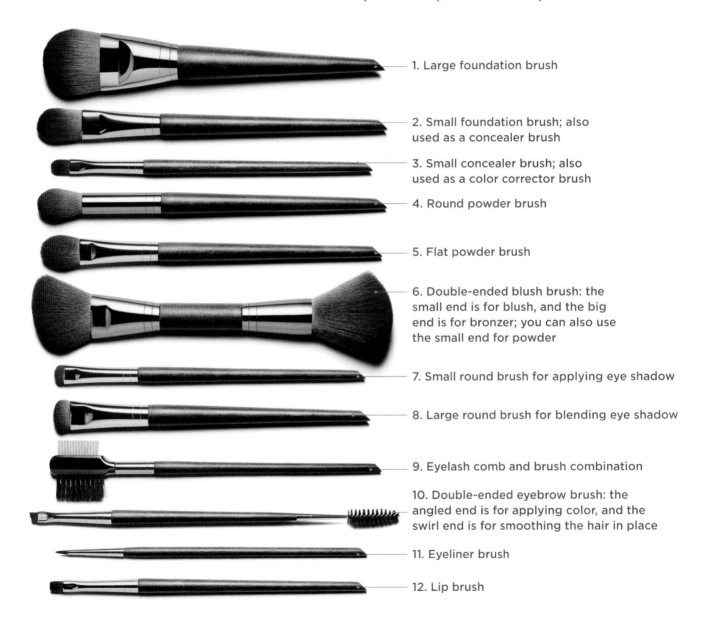

1. Large foundation brush

2. Small foundation brush; also used as a concealer brush

3. Small concealer brush; also used as a color corrector brush

4. Round powder brush

5. Flat powder brush

6. Double-ended blush brush: the small end is for blush, and the big end is for bronzer; you can also use the small end for powder

7. Small round brush for applying eye shadow

8. Large round brush for blending eye shadow

9. Eyelash comb and brush combination

10. Double-ended eyebrow brush: the angled end is for applying color, and the swirl end is for smoothing the hair in place

11. Eyeliner brush

12. Lip brush

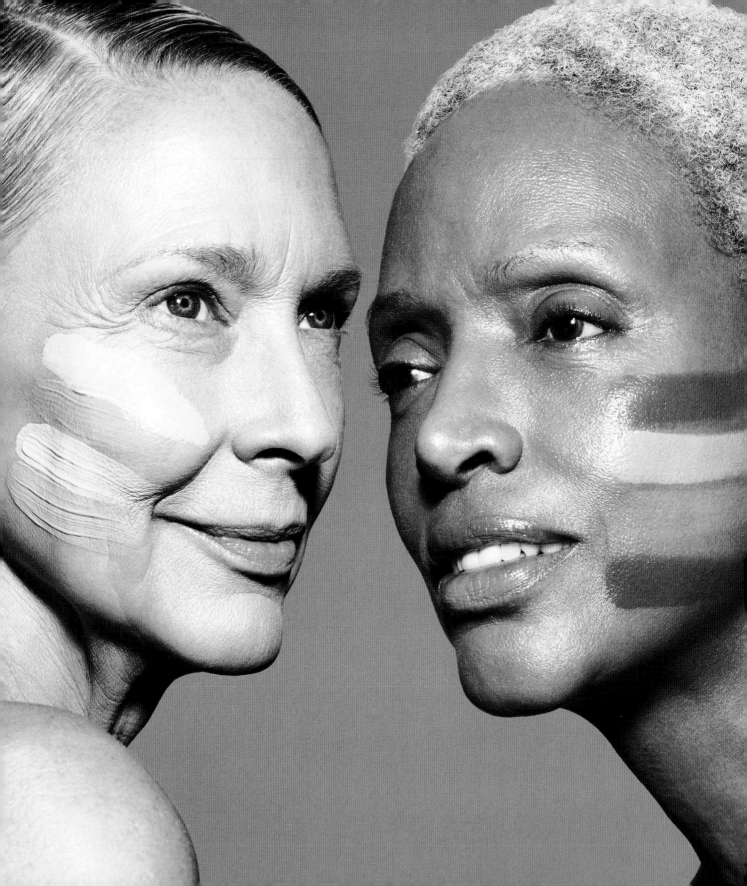

3 FOUNDATION

For some women, the word "foundation" already sounds like too much makeup. Maybe that's because many years back, foundation was thicker than it is today and gave the skin a cakey look that made the wearer appear older. However, today's foundations are more lightweight, meaning that you can wear them and still look youthful, dewy, and natural.

WHAT *NOT* TO BUY WHEN SHOPPING FOR FOUNDATION

- Skip all foundation meant for combination or oily skin, including mattifying foundation, oil-free foundation, pressed-powder foundation, and mineral formulas. Those will only make your skin look dry.

- Most stick foundation is also way too heavy for mature skin.

- CC creams—or color-correcting creams—contain too many chemicals, and the result is a masklike appearance. They might look good in TV commercial lighting, but in real life, they're too heavy.

- BB creams—or blemish-balm creams—are also not great for maturing women.

- Don't believe advertising that promotes a foundation's "lifting, firming, and antiaging" qualities. Foundation is not a skincare product: makeup simply can't nourish your skin.

CHOOSING THE RIGHT WEIGHT

Because skin becomes dry as we age, foundation should be hydrating and not too heavy. Light foundation is easy and quick to apply and matches your skin color more easily than heavy foundation. Because there are thousands of foundations out there, let's concentrate on the best choices: tinted moisturizers and hydrating liquid foundations.

Tinted moisturizer

Tinted moisturizer has the lightest weight of any type of makeup base. I like it because it gives the most natural, radiant result and is perfect for dry skin. It doesn't give you much coverage, so you will want to use concealer in the corners of your eyes, on your eyelids, and in any other areas that need touch-ups. You can apply tinted moisturizer with your fingers. Remember to blend downward toward your neck. It is a more natural way of blending the tinted moisturizer (or foundation) on your neck, and it blends better in this direction.

Lightweight hydrating foundation

This is my choice for an everyday go-to foundation because it feels natural and evens out your complexion but offers more coverage than tinted moisturizer. You can apply it with your fingers, a foundation brush, or a latex-free sponge.

Medium-weight hydrating foundation

This provides more coverage than lightweight foundation and is ideal if you have skin conditions such as rosacea or sun spots. Use a foundation brush, a sponge, or your fingers to apply it. Follow up the application by lightly powdering your eyelids, the under-eye area, the middle of the forehead, and around the nose for a matte finish.

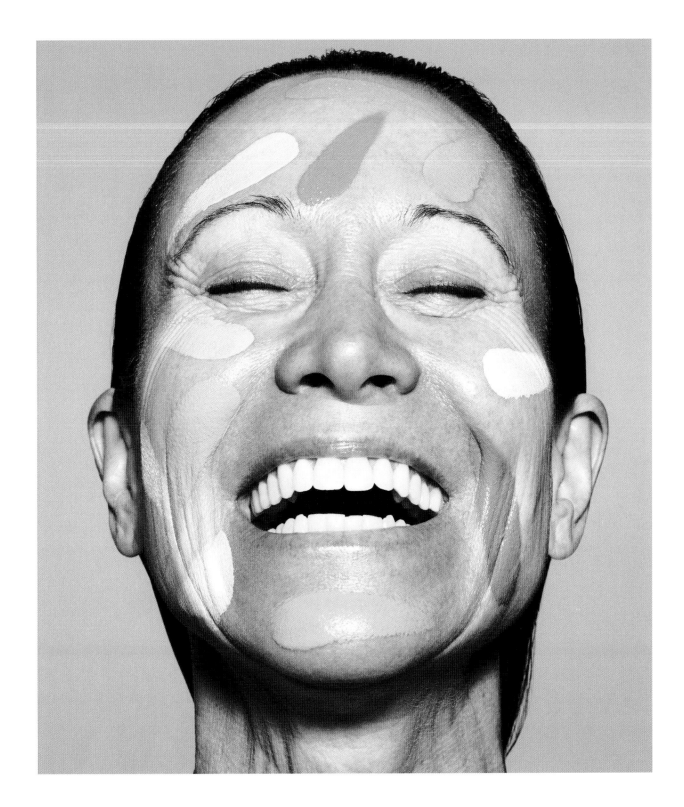

CHOOSING THE RIGHT COLOR

Knowing the undertone of your skin makes choosing the right foundation much easier. You don't want your makeup looking too light, dark, ashy, or muddy. The right color really wakes up your whole face!

- If you have cool undertones, your skin is pinkish or bluish, especially if your complexion is light. I recommend a yellow-based foundation because aging skin often looks a bit gray, so the hint of yellow gives life back to the face. Avoid all pink-based foundations.

- If you have warm undertones, your skin is yellowish and golden, so choose a foundation from the warm-toned family.

- If your undertone is neutral, without much pink or yellow, it might be a challenge to find a matching foundation. Many cosmetics companies won't offer colors that match your face and neck exactly. If that's the case for you, then buy two different colors and mix them.

BUYING THE FOUNDATION

If you are not accustomed to using and buying foundation, I recommend reading the latest reviews in beauty magazines or on beauty blogs aimed at mature women. Then go to a store where you can test the products. Ask the sales professionals or makeup artists to apply the products to your face, then ask their opinion. Ask them to show you how to use concealer. Look in the mirror while the makeup artist is working and ask questions. The color should match perfectly: there should be no color difference between your face and neck.

After the makeup is done, step outside with a hand mirror and look at your face in the daylight. It's the right foundation for you if it looks natural, the color matches perfectly, and it feels like you're not wearing any makeup.

Apply foundation after performing your morning skincare routine (toner, serum, moisturizer, and sunblock). You always want to wait ten to fifteen minutes for all the skincare products to absorb before moving on to the foundation. If it is simply lying on top of the sunscreen, it might peel off.

CONCEALER

If you don't want to wear any makeup at all, try using just concealer. It is a real miracle worker—it can hide tired eyes, discoloration, rosacea, and light sun spots. Concealer should be in the same color family as your foundation, only a half shade lighter.

Apply it after the foundation—you might find you need less because your foundation has already covered some of the problem areas. Use a small concealer brush or your ring finger to dab it on. A little goes a long way!

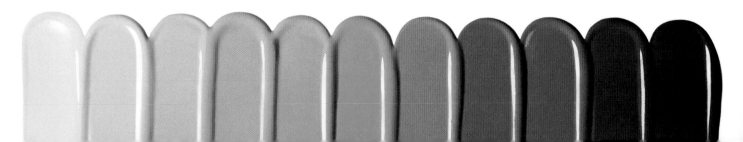

Seal the concealer with a light dusting of powder to prevent it from running off your face during the course of the day.

COLOR CORRECTOR

High-pigmentation color correctors allow you to hide areas on your face that your foundation or concealer can't cover, including heavy rosacea, dark circles around the eyes, birthmarks, redness, and dark sun spots.

You can use a color corrector under concealer and foundation. But you must add a loose or compact powder after the color corrector, concealer, and foundation are all applied to set them.

Light skin: Use yellow to neutralize any purple undertones and conceal veins and redness; use lavender to neutralize any yellow undertones

Light skin: Use olive green to conceal broken capillaries

Light skin: Use peach to neutralize any blue undertones and cover brown spots and sun spots

Medium or tan skin: Use dark peach to neutralize any olive-gray undertones

Dark skin: Use brick to neutralize any gray undertones

Dark skin: Use caramel to cover dark spots, scars, and pigmentation marks

Very dark skin: Use orange to neutralize any dark areas around the mouth and forehead

Very dark skin: Use deep brown to darken and neutralize any light and depigmented areas

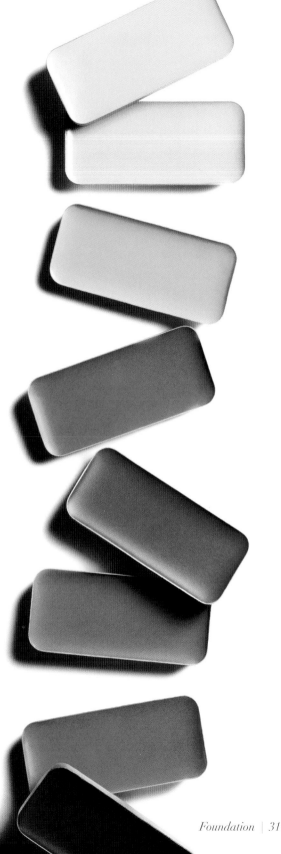

POWDER

Powder is almost a curse for mature women because it can make the skin look dry. But you need a light touch of powder around the eyes, on top of concealer and color corrector, and on your T-zone (your forehead, nose, and chin) in order to keep these products in place. You can use pressed or loose powders applied with a small powder brush. Be very light-handed.

The right powder color, like the right foundation color, is very important. For light skin, transparent powder is best. For medium skin, use a yellow-based powder, and for dark skin, use a peach-orange powder.

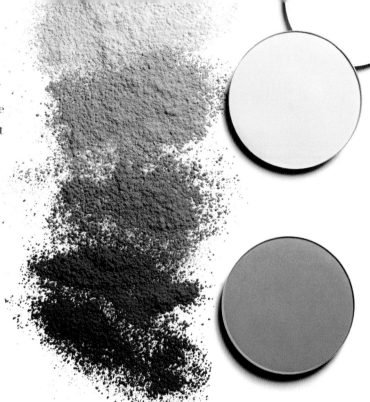

PRIMERS: EYELID PRIMER AND FACE PRIMER

Eyelid primer is a must to keep eye shadow on your lids. It is designed to prevent powdered eye shadows from creasing. Just tap it onto your ring finger, then tap it onto your lids up to the brow bone and blend well. Apply your concealer or foundation on top of that, finish with just a hint of powder, and the base for your long-lasting eye shadow is ready!

You do not need face primer during the day because your skin has already been prepped by your skincare products. Your serum and hydrating moisturizer already give you a smooth surface for the foundation. But I recommend using face primer for evening makeup, right after your serum and moisturizer. When choosing a primer, make sure it does not contain dimethicone, a silicon-based polymer that is not good for mature skin.

How to Apply Foundation to Various Skin Tones

VERY LIGHT SKIN *Maarit*

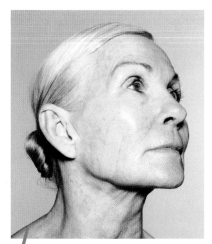

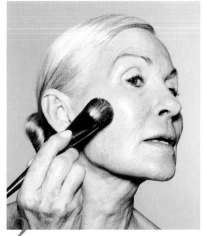

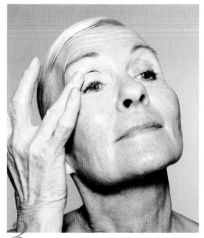

1. Choose a foundation that matches your neck perfectly, so it works on your face as well.

2. Apply foundation with a large foundation brush (#1 on page 25) all over the face, then blend into the neck.

3. Apply concealer to the lids. If you don't have dark circles under your eyes, concealer is not necessary there.

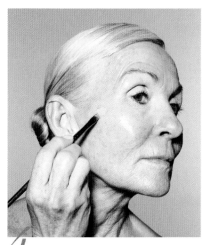

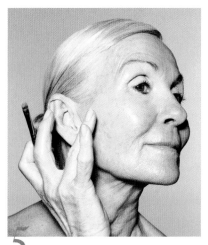

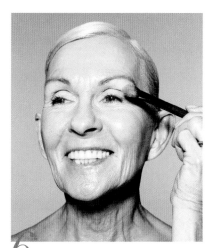

4. Use a brush to apply concealer to any light sun spots.

5. Use your ring finger to pat concealer on any big sun spots.

6. Lightly apply transparent loose powder on the eyelids, under the eyes, around the nose, and in the middle of the forehead.

LIGHT SKIN *Tamiyo*

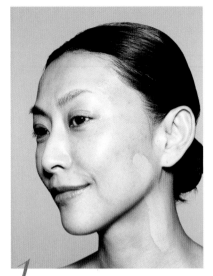

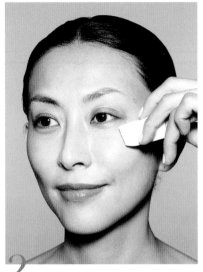

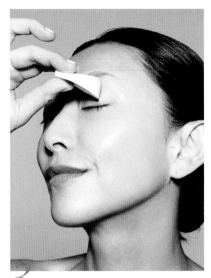

1. Choose a foundation that matches your skin and neck.

2. Dip a latex-free triangle-shaped sponge in your foundation and tap the sponge onto your face. Blend evenly.

3. Apply foundation to the eyelids as well.

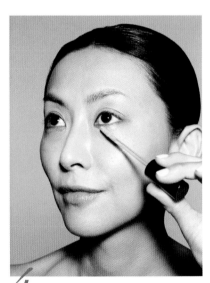

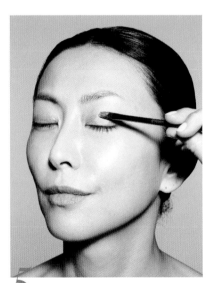

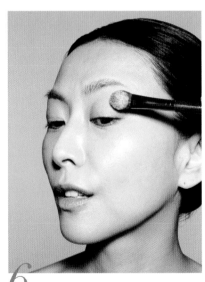

4. Apply concealer under the eyes if you have dark circles.

5. Use a concealer brush to apply concealer to the lids as well.

6. To get super-dewy skin, powder the eyelids and under the eyes only, not the T-zone.

TAN SKIN *Elizabeth*

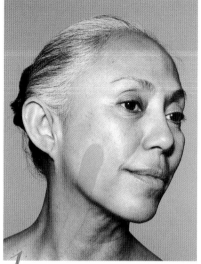

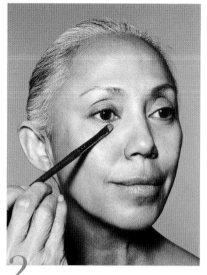

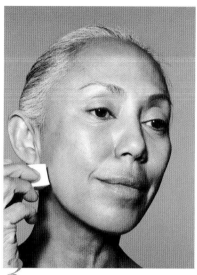

1. Make sure the foundation you choose blends well with your face and neck. Elizabeth's face is one degree lighter than her neck and body, so I needed to darken her face with a darker foundation to match.

2. Use a peach color corrector, applied with a concealer brush, to hide dark under-eye circles.

3. Use a latex-free triangle-shaped sponge to tap the foundation onto your skin.

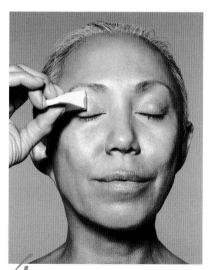

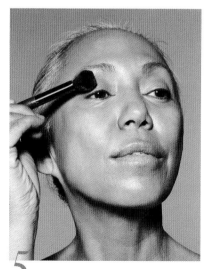

4. Apply foundation to the eyelids as well.

5. Use a round powder brush (#4 on page 25) to apply loose powder on the eyelids, under the eye, and on the T-zone.

DARK SKIN *Coco*

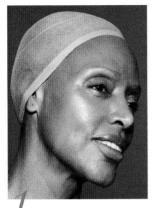

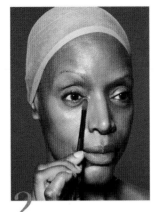

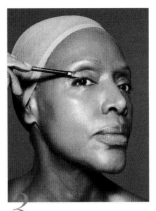

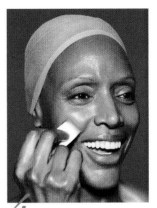

1. Choose a light yellow-orange foundation to match golden undertones in the skin and neck.

2. Using a concealer brush, apply orange color corrector to the inner corners of the eyes.

3. Add color corrector to the eyelids.

4. Use a latex-free triangle-shaped sponge to tap the foundation onto your skin.

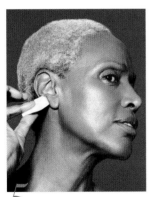

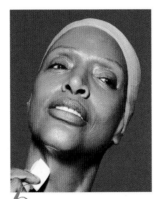

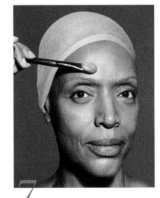

5. If you have short hair, remember to apply a bit of foundation to your ears.

6. Blend the foundation onto your neck.

7. Apply loose powder to the T-zone as well as to the eyelids.

VERY DARK SKIN *Ebony*

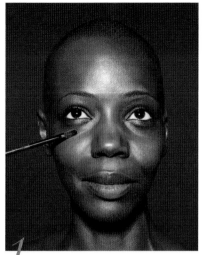

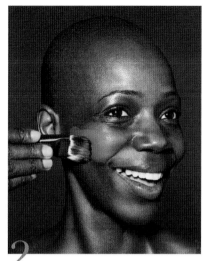

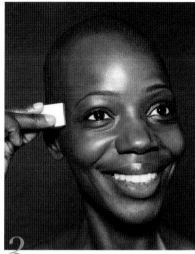

1. Using a concealer brush and/ or your finger, apply a deep orange color corrector around the eyes to wash out any dark discolorations.

2. Choose an orange-based foundation to really bring out a dark complexion. Use a large foundation brush to apply it.

3. Use a latex-free triangle-shaped sponge to tap the foundation onto the skin. Blend well.

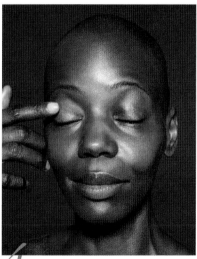

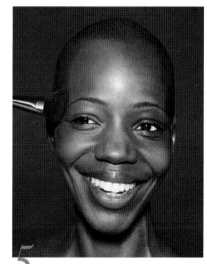

4. Lightly tap loose powder onto eyelids.

5. If your skin is still oily, lightly apply loose powder with the large end of a double-ended blush brush (#6 on page 25) all around the face, including the eyelids and under the eyes.

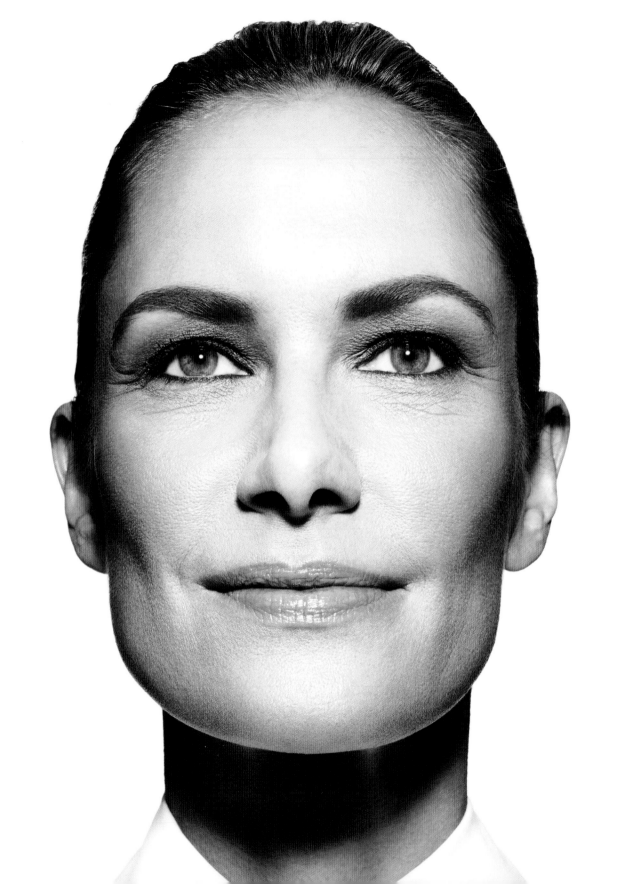

4

BLUSH

If there is one makeup product that will give you a lift and wake up your entire face, it is blush.

CREAM BLUSH

I like to use cream blush on mature women because it looks the most natural, glides on smoothly, blends perfectly, and gives the cheeks an amazing sheen. Cream blush gives your face a real lift, whereas powdered blush brings out your fine lines. Cream blush is always applied on bare skin or on top of your tinted moisturizer or foundation and concealer, if used.

Dark skin looks great with a bright coral blush (as on Coco, top right). Apply it with a latex-free triangle-shaped sponge for the best result. Tap the sponge on the back of your hand first to get rid of excess blush, and make sure you don't apply too much to your face. Swipe the blush on the apples of your cheeks and tap it upward to the hairline, then use the sponge's clean side to blend and smooth.

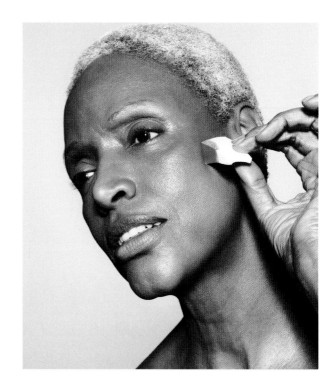

Model Gunilla Lindblad (bottom right) uses a sponge to apply blush: she taps the product on her skin, then blends it so there aren't any lines of demarcation. When she's finished, she looks like she was just blushing!

I asked Gunilla, 72, about her beauty routine and philosophy. She works as a New York City guide and was one of the first Swedish supermodels in the late 1960s and 1970s.

What makeup products do you use?

I wear makeup only when I work, and then it is mostly on my eyes: pencil liner and mascara. I have always curled my lashes to open my eyes. When I was modeling, the great French makeup artist Thibault

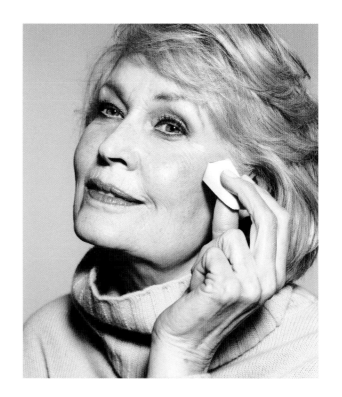

Vabre curled my lashes with a teaspoon, which he did for his private client Catherine Deneuve as well. I also use a cream blush.

What is the most important message about beauty that you want to convey to younger generations?

For all women of my generation and generations to come: cultivate beautiful, glowing skin. Mix a few drops of rose-hip oil with your moisturizer. Highlight your eyes, and always know less is more.

RIKU'S TIPS

- Always apply blush to the apples of the cheeks, then blend well, outward and upward, for the most natural result. Find the apples of your cheeks by smiling.

- The best colors for almost any kind of skin are shades of pink, from the lightest salmon pink to the brightest fuchsia and darkest berry. The lighter your skin, the lighter your blush should be, and vice versa. Also, sienna, peach, and coral shades work throughout the year for darker skin.

Top to bottom:

Cream blush
Powdered blush
Bronzer

POWDERED BLUSH

Use powdered blush if your skin is oily, because cream blush doesn't last a long time on the skin when oil pushes through makeup. Powdered blush is also a good choice if you want your cheeks to look less dewy and have a more matte finish.

- Make sure to use powdered blush only on top of your tinted moisturizer or foundation and powdered cheeks. If you don't powder your cheeks first, the blush won't glide on smoothly.

- When you're ready, dip a blush brush into the product, then swirl it in the palm of your hand to remove any excess.

- Tap the brush on the apples of the cheeks and start blending right away so the color is concentrated on the plumpest part of the cheeks and fades upward toward the tragus (the little bump of cartilage in front of the ear). You can also use a latex-free triangle-shaped sponge to blend.

- Blend well, so there are no lines of demarcation.

- If you applied too much blush, tap a small amount of loose powder on top of the blush to make it fade a little.

BRONZER

Light sand and cinnamon bronzer provide enough color for light skin, while women who have tan and dark skin should use colors such as deep gold, terracotta, and deep cinnamon.

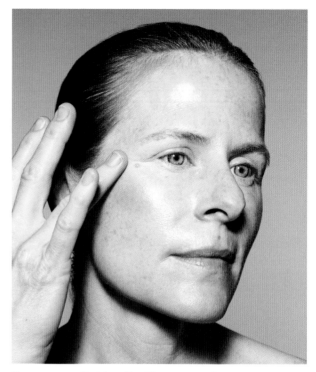

Teresa uses light-reflecting cream bronzer (without shimmer), which she applies and blends on her cheeks with her fingers.

Cream bronzer gives you a healthful, radiant, sun-kissed result. I like stick bronzers, which are easy to use and travel well. If your skin is very dry, choose a cream bronzer and apply it just as you would blush. I recommend using a latex-free triangle-shaped sponge to apply the product on top of tinted moisturizer or foundation.

If you prefer a powdered bronzer, choose a matte variety that doesn't contain any light-reflecting prisms: the particles get stuck on your skin, making fine lines and wrinkles stand out and making your skin look older. And nobody likes that! Use your blush brush and apply it exactly the same way you would apply powdered blush.

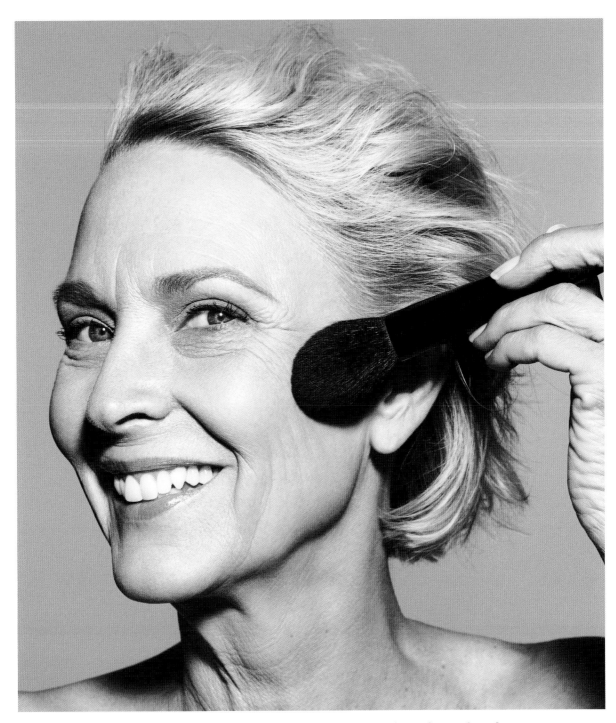

Model Karen Bjornson applies pink powdered blush on the apples of her cheeks. She smiles to find the correct place for the blush.

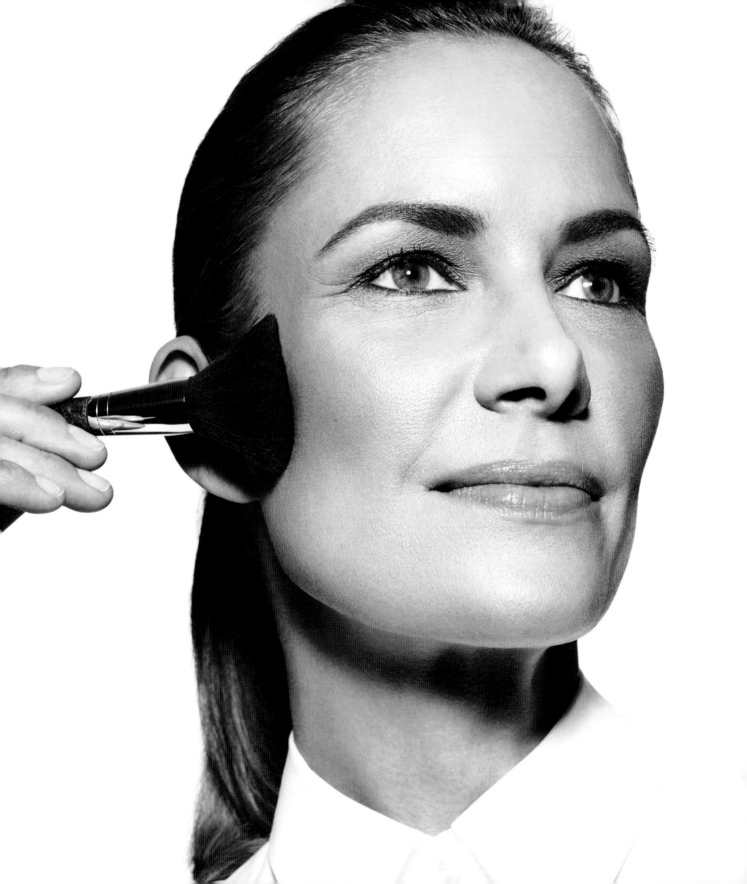

CONTOURING

Contouring your face does not really work when you're over 40. It looks good under spotlights at red-carpet events, on reality TV shows, and on catwalks, but in real life, you can end up looking like you're trying way too hard and wearing tons of stage makeup—à la Joan Collins.

For evening makeup, you can use a little matte bronzer to contour your cheeks, but don't overdo it.

Don't use bronzer to contour your cheeks during the daytime. It drags your face down and looks too made-up.

Left: Model Allison Walton contours her cheeks with bronzer in preparation for applying her evening makeup.

HIGHLIGHTER

I love metallic liquid highlighters, which really bring your cheeks to life. Again, do not use highlighters that contain visible glitter or prisms. Use a latex-free triangle-shaped sponge to apply them to your skin by tapping and blending the product on top of tinted moisturizer or foundation.

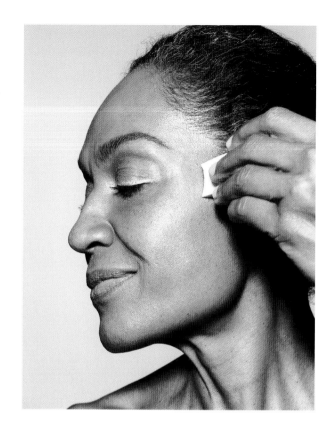

Light gold and pink-champagne look good on light skin; gold, copper, and bronze shades look good on tan and dark skin. Avoid other colors—they will end up looking too frosty.

Above: Model Pat Tracey uses a sponge to apply highlighter to her cheeks. A small amount goes a long way!

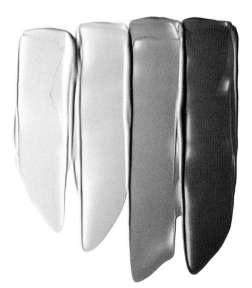

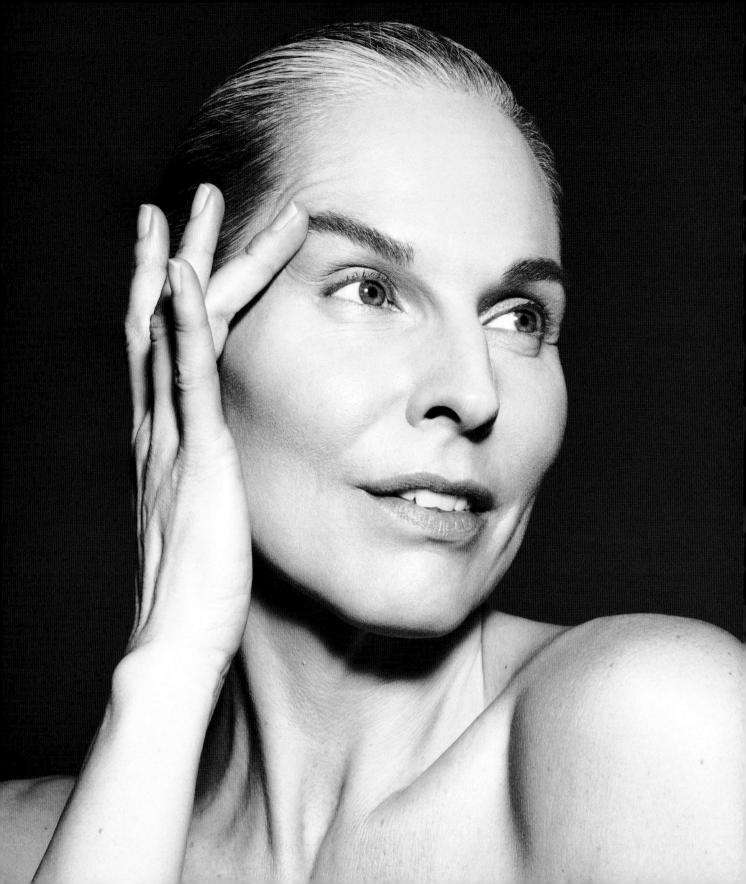

5 EYEBROWS

Eyebrows are sometimes overrated: they shouldn't be the main focus of your makeup. Some women—including actress Whoopi Goldberg and model Kristen McMenamy—have almost no eyebrows at all, and they look cool like that because it's their style. Other women—including actresses Julia Roberts, Brooke Shields, and Sofia Vergara—have made lush eyebrows their natural trademark. Even the late great Mexican painter Frida Kahlo's unibrow came to define her look.

What looks best on one person doesn't necessarily look best on another. Eyebrow styles depend on your overall style: your hair color, haircut, clothing, bone structure, and makeup. Also, we know that as we get older, the brows get thinner and more uneven and sometimes turn gray. Fortunately, there are many ways to make your eyebrows look more youthful.

If you're not sure how to shape and trim your brows, ask an aesthetician or brow-bar professional. She or he will teach you how to neaten your brow area yourself with the help of tweezers, brow razors, and brow scissors.

Next, I will show you a variety of ways to enhance your brows. And always, always, always remember: when choosing a brow-makeup color, choose one a shade lighter than or the same color as your natural brows.

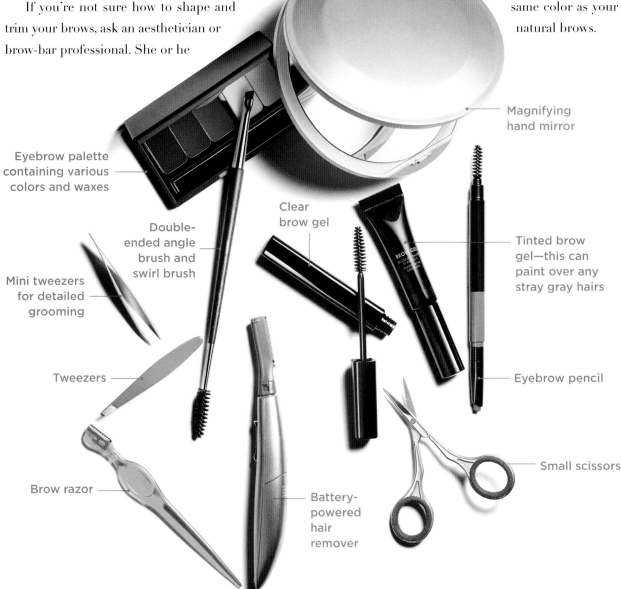

Eyebrow palette containing various colors and waxes

Double-ended angle brush and swirl brush

Mini tweezers for detailed grooming

Tweezers

Brow razor

Clear brow gel

Battery-powered hair remover

Magnifying hand mirror

Tinted brow gel—this can paint over any stray gray hairs

Eyebrow pencil

Small scissors

HOW TO STYLE YOUR EYEBROWS

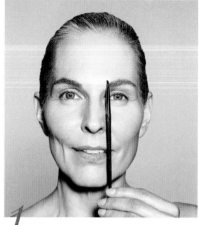

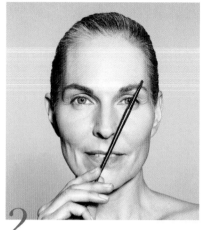

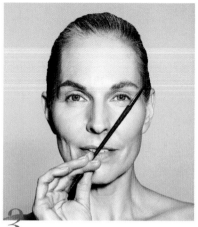

1. Place an eyebrow brush or pencil on one side of your nose and point it straight up toward your brows: this is where your brows should start. Anything between that point and your other eyebrow should be tweezed or shaved.

2. Leaving the brush at the side of your nose, point it diagonally from your nostril to the outside edge of your iris: this is where your brows should arch.

3. Point your brush from the outside corner of your nose diagonally to the outside corner of your eye: this is where your brows should end.

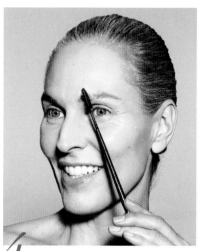

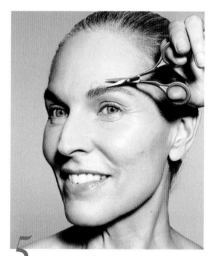

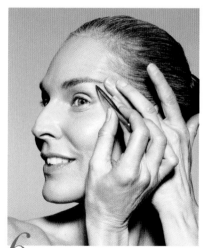

4. Brush your brows against their growing direction so you can see any long hairs that need to be trimmed.

5. Using brow scissors, trim your brows very carefully: just take off a very small amount at the top, so your natural shape still exists.

6. Using tweezers, clean any hair under the brows that doesn't belong on the brow line. Stretch your skin with your other hand to give yourself a flat and tight surface for tweezing (it is also less painful that way). Always tweeze *with* the hair's natural growing direction.

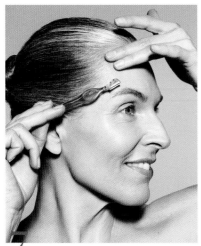

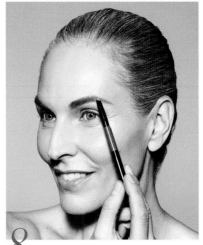

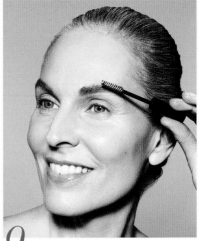

7. Use a brow shaver to trim any hair around the brows: it is fast, safe, and completely painless.

8. Apply color to the brows by filling them in with a pencil in small strokes — this will make the result look most natural. Be sure to powder the brow area before you fill in your brows, especially if you have oily or combination skin, as it will help set a base that will keep everything in place. Instead of using a pencil to fill in the brows, you can also dip the angled end of the eyebrow brush into powder and brush it into your brows. As for color, I like to choose something that matches the color of your hair (if your hair is black, choose more of a dark gray, which will look smoother).

9. Finish with a brow gel, which will set every hair in place and give your brows a beautiful sheen.

After she's finished, model MaryAnn Elizabeth's brows blend with the rest of her makeup and don't overpower her face. The look is very classic and elegant.

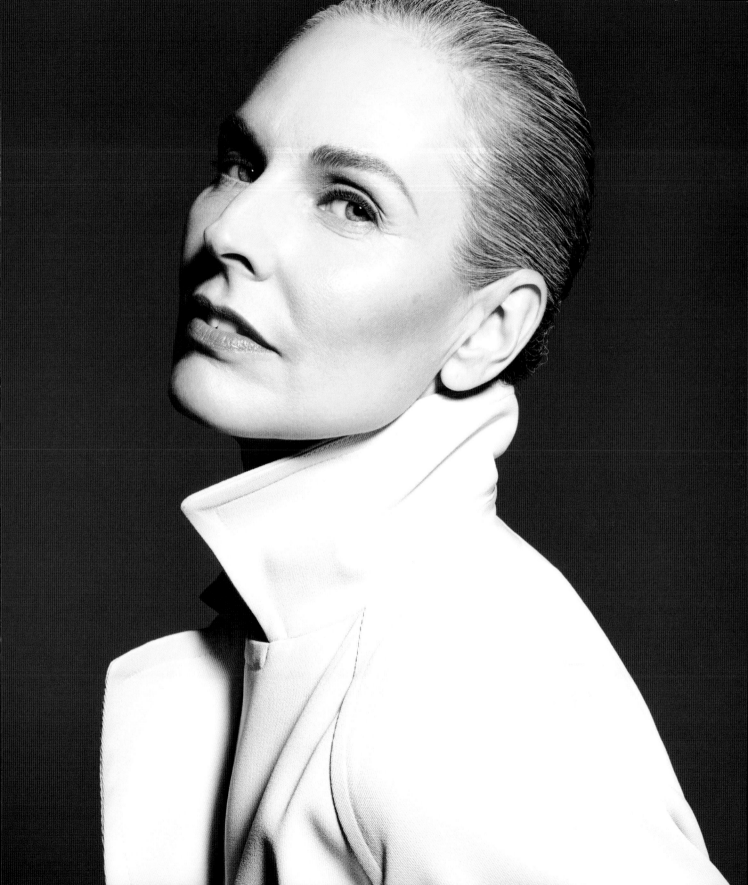

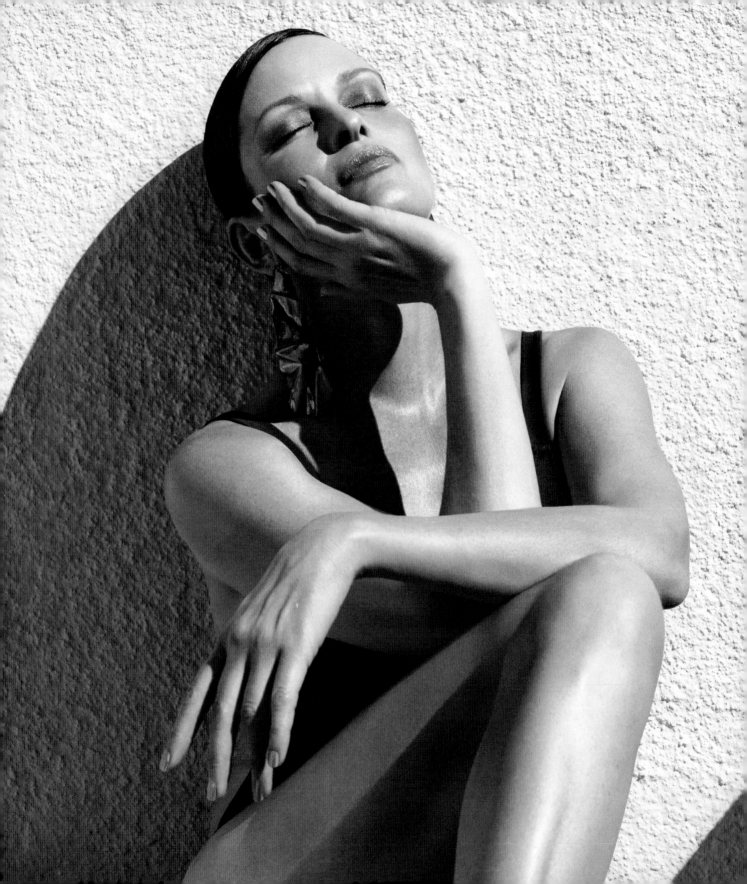

PERMANENT AND SEMIPERMANENT OPTIONS

EYEBROW TINTING

Eyebrow tinting is the easiest way to give your brows a little lift. The most important thing is to choose the right color: never go too dark, because it makes your eyes look tired and drags them down. I recommend choosing the color closest to your natural brow color: a gray-brown mix works well for fair and gray hair, and a gray-black mix works well for dark hair. The tint lasts around a month.

EYEBROW TATTOO

I am not a big fan of eyebrow tattoos, because quite often they look too drawn-on and theatrical. Over time, the coloring can change, too, making the brows turn blue-green and even orange-yellow. The ink is permanent, so if you do choose this option, make sure your tattoo artist has a website that includes before-and-after images so you can really see her or his work. It is very important to make sure you will be happy with the result because it will be there for a lifetime.

MICROBLADING

Microblading involves the application of a special pigment via individual hairlike strokes. The result is designed to look natural, like real hair. The pigment lasts one to two years before it starts to fade. Again, choosing a technician is very important, so do your homework and check out her or his website or Instagram page. Look for a portfolio that shows before-and-after images.

The results vary. Some women swear by microblading, and some are disappointed. It's like trying a new hair color—you might love it, you might not.

The last thing you want is for your tattooed or microbladed eyebrows to be the focus of your face. That doesn't look good on anyone and can make you look older.

EYEBROW GROWTH SERUMS

Eyebrow growth serums help new hair grow and might give your brows a fuller look. But you must continue using the product to maintain growth.

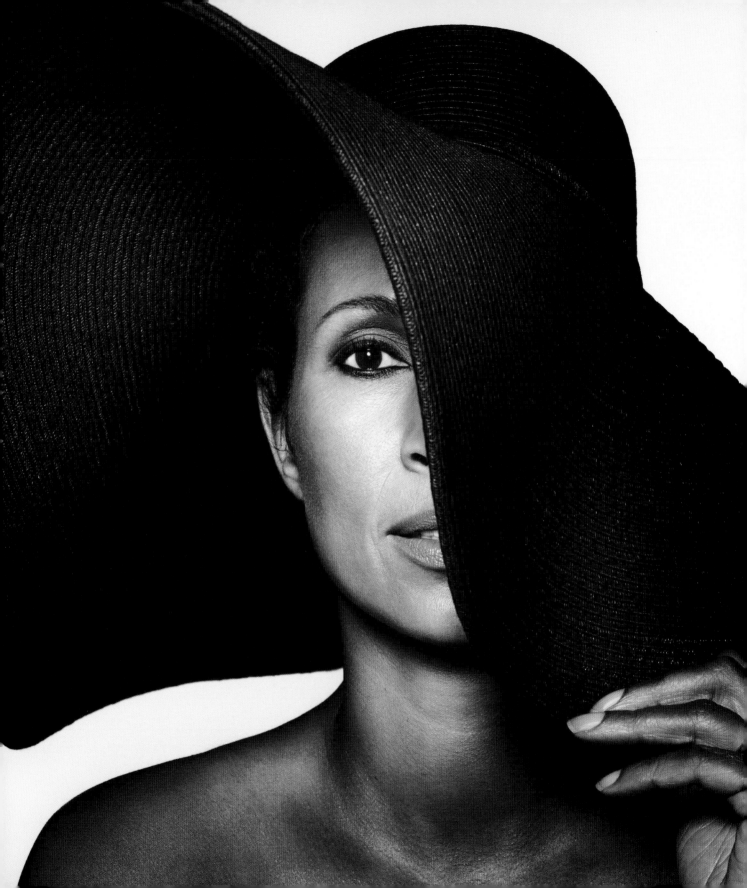

6 EYE SHADOW

For lots of women, the most challenging part of makeup is applying eye shadow. The questions I often hear are:

- Which colors are best for mature women?

- How do I apply eye shadow correctly?

- What kinds of brushes do I need?

RIKU'S TIPS

- Powdered eye shadows are best for mature women because they stay a long time on the lids and don't crease as easily as cream eye shadows.

- For daytime use, eye shadow finishes should be matte. Glittery or sparkling eye shadows reflect light with a shimmer power that brings out the fine lines on your eyelids and around your eyes. And that you don't want.

- For evening use, you can choose a light-reflecting shadow, but don't choose anything that contains glitter or light-reflecting prisms. They look too obvious and get stuck in your lines, calling attention to them.

- You can use just one color or go with two to three colors or add even more! If you're not sure what looks best, stick with earthy, neutral colors.

- On *very light* and *light skin*, taupe and light brown work well.

- On *tan skin*, go for terra-cotta, golden brown, and dark peach. Women with tan skin should avoid pastels and light grays and browns because they look ashy and dull.

- On *very dark* and *ebony skin*, use deep terra-cotta, matte bronze, and burgundy, or go for bold colors such as bright purple, green, and blue. Dark navy blue always looks amazing on a smoky eye. Avoid white and pastels because they can look ashy on your skin.

First of all, you can use just one eye shadow or as many as you want or none at all. There are no rules about how many colors you can and cannot use. It all depends on what kind of eye makeup you like most. One woman likes to use a single neutral matte eye shadow; another likes navy blue and black. It also depends on your personal style: you can make it simple and minimalist or go bold and colorful or do anything in between.

My techniques for applying eye makeup all are very simple, and you can learn the basics quickly. I recommend that you purchase a matte palette containing three basic colors:

- a light color that is applied on the entire lid up to the crease,

- a medium-dark color that creates a shadow on the crease and the lash line, and

- a dark color that creates a shadow by the lashes or is used as a liner. This color is appropriate for evening makeup.

Daytime and Evening Eye Shadow

Following are examples of very basic daytime and evening eye shadow techniques demonstrated by model Marni Malinosky, who is 51. Before applying eye shadow, be sure to apply eyelid primer all over the lids as well as concealer, foundation, and a little powder (see page 32).

NUDE LOOK

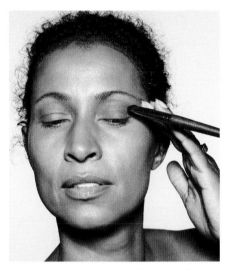

If you want a super-simple, natural-looking, and fast eye shadow technique, use just one color on the lids and no mascara. Use a brush to apply light terra-cotta matte eye shadow all over the lids, up to the crease. The color will go a bit over the crease when you blend it in.

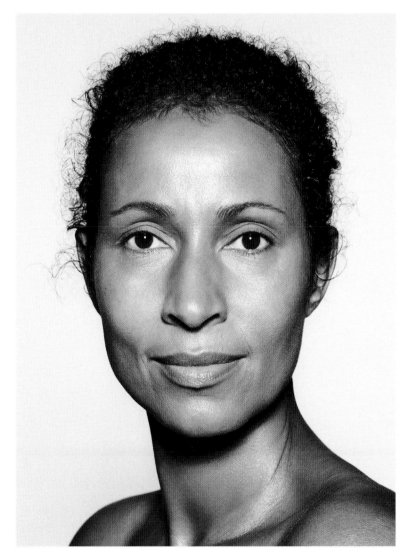

WITH POWDERED LINER AND MASCARA

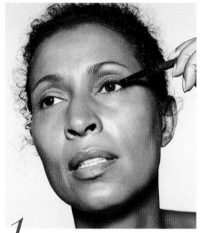 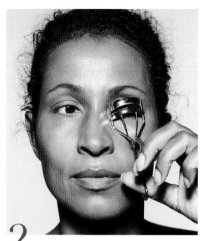 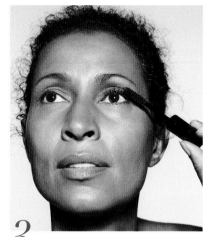

1. Use dark eye shadow as a liner. Apply it with a small eye shadow brush (#7 on page 25) on your lash line and blend.

2. Curl your lashes.

3. Brush on black waterproof mascara.

WITH POWDERED LINER ON LOWER LASHES

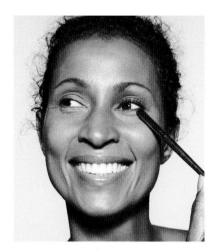 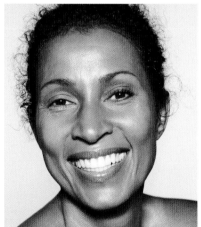

Apply the same dark eye shadow just below your bottom lashes, and your eyes will pop out a little more. The liner accentuates the shape of your eyes.

To turn this into an evening look, you just need to add a few simple steps.

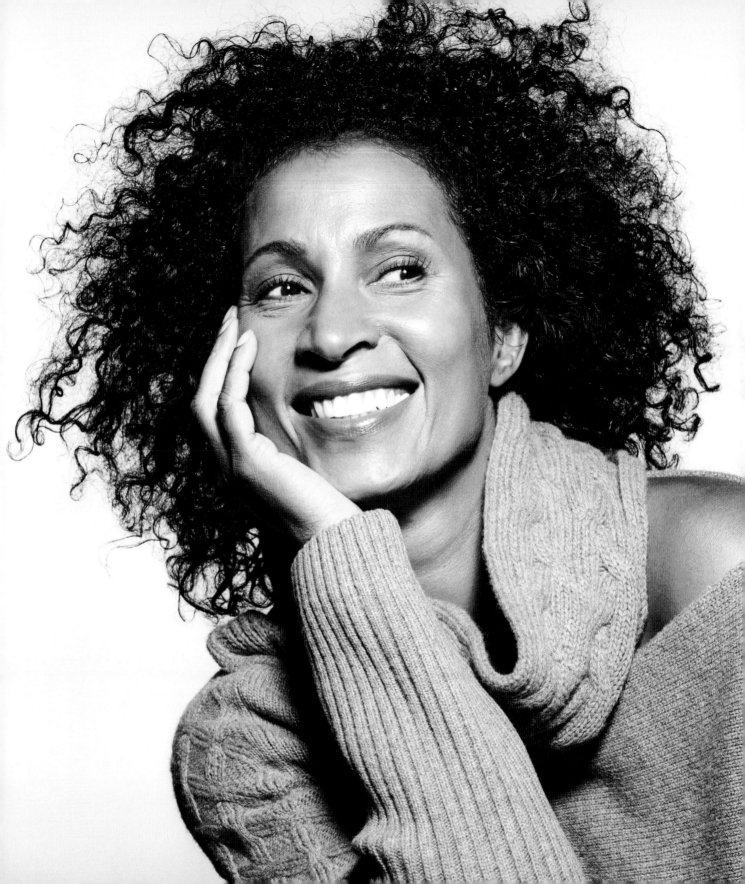

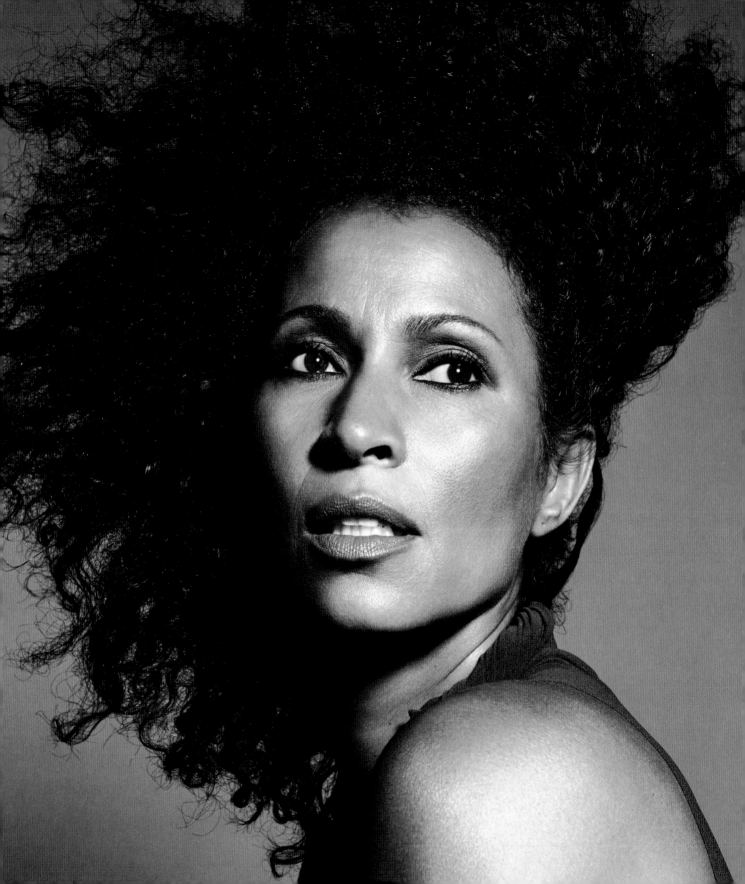

WITH LIFTING EFFECT ON THE CREASE

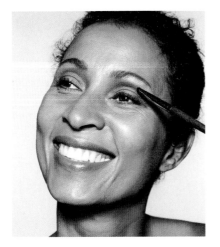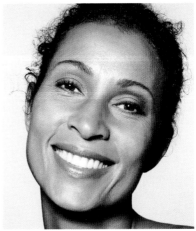

Extend the dark eye shadow from the inner to the outer corners of the eyes, right along the crease. Your eyes will look bigger, and the shadow will seem to lift the eyes.

WITH EYELINER

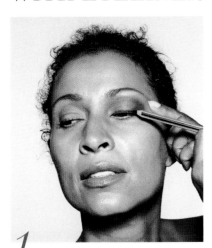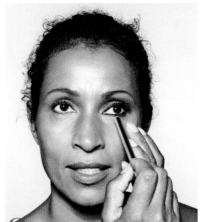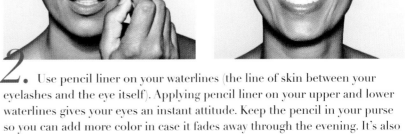

1. Use pencil liner on the upper lash line: black really brings the eyes out. Blend the line with a small round brush (#7 on page 25) to soften.

2. Use pencil liner on your waterlines (the line of skin between your eyelashes and the eye itself). Applying pencil liner on your upper and lower waterlines gives your eyes an instant attitude. Keep the pencil in your purse so you can add more color in case it fades away through the evening. It's also a good idea to keep a couple of cotton swabs in your purse for touch-ups.

EYELINER MASTER CLASS

If you are not an eye shadow lady, you can just use an eye pencil and mascara, which will bring your eyes out beautifully. Pencil liners come in amazing color variations, so you don't always have to stick to black and dark brown. How about navy blue or dark green for the daytime and cobalt blue or gold for the evening? The textures vary from matte to shimmery. Metallic liners work well on mature skin, but avoid pencils that have glitter in them.

- Waterproof pencils last longer because the eyes of mature women tend to water. They dry fast, so you must blend and soften the line right after you apply it.

- White pencil liner on your waterline always brightens your eyes and makes them look bigger.

- Dark pencils on the waterline shrink your eyes. I like to use dark pencils on the waterline because they lift the eyes and make them really pop.

- Basic colors, like black and dark chocolate brown, always work. Brown makes the eyes look softer than black and dark navy blue.

- If you don't like pencils, you can use dark matte eye shadow as an eyeliner. It blends well and always looks soft. Use your eye shadow brush to apply and blend it.

- Liquid eyeliner is the most challenging to apply. You might already be a master at the technique, but if not, you need to practice. The line must be solid and straight on the lash line.

- The best eyeliner medium is gel because it glides more easily, gives a softer result, and is easier to apply than liquid eyeliner. If you make a mistake with gel liner, it's easy to fix. See the Hollywood Glamour and Classic Glamour makeovers (pages 155 and 189) for specific guidelines.

Eye Shadow with Karen

I want to show you two different looks that incorporate the basic eye shadow technique I've just explained.

My model is Karen Bjornson, 68, who was a model and muse for the legendary fashion designer Halston. Karen has always placed a high priority on good health, which has allowed her to age gracefully from the inside out.

What daily beauty routines do you never skip?

Sunscreen is a must. And before that, I wash my face and apply face serum and face oil.

What beauty wisdom have you imparted to your children?

I have two beautiful daughters, and I asked them what they remember. They both said that I always told them to use sunscreen, curl their lashes, and put on mascara.

What does beauty mean to you?

Beauty is a thing that takes your breath away. It can be a flower, a sunset, or a woman walking into a room.

How has the meaning of beauty changed for you through the years?

In my 20s, I worked with some of the most beautiful people in fashion in New York City, but now that I'm 68, beauty has a much deeper meaning. It is the whole person, not the shell. Now I believe that beauty comes from intellect, confidence, kindness, humor, and overall style.

What makes you feel beautiful?

When my husband compliments me on how I look or what I am wearing.

What is your motto for life?

Find the magic every day.

DAY LOOK

Here I show you how to create a very basic look that lifts your eyes and brings them out. This look works also as more natural evening makeup. Be sure to prep your eyelids with eyelid primer and foundation (see page 32).

1. Apply light brown matte eye shadow along the lash line to create depth. Right after you have applied the color, blend it so it looks soft.

2. Apply the same light brown on the crease, which creates a shadow that lifts your eyes and makes them look bigger. Blend well with a blending brush—back and forth like a windshield wiper—until the shadow looks soft and natural.

3. Curl the lashes.

4. Apply mascara.

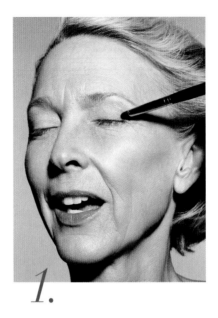

1.

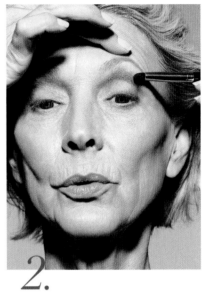

2.

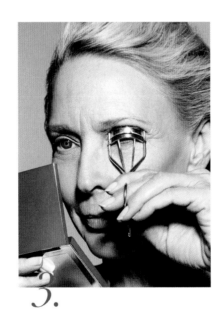

3.

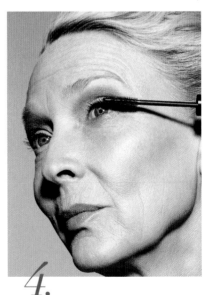

4.

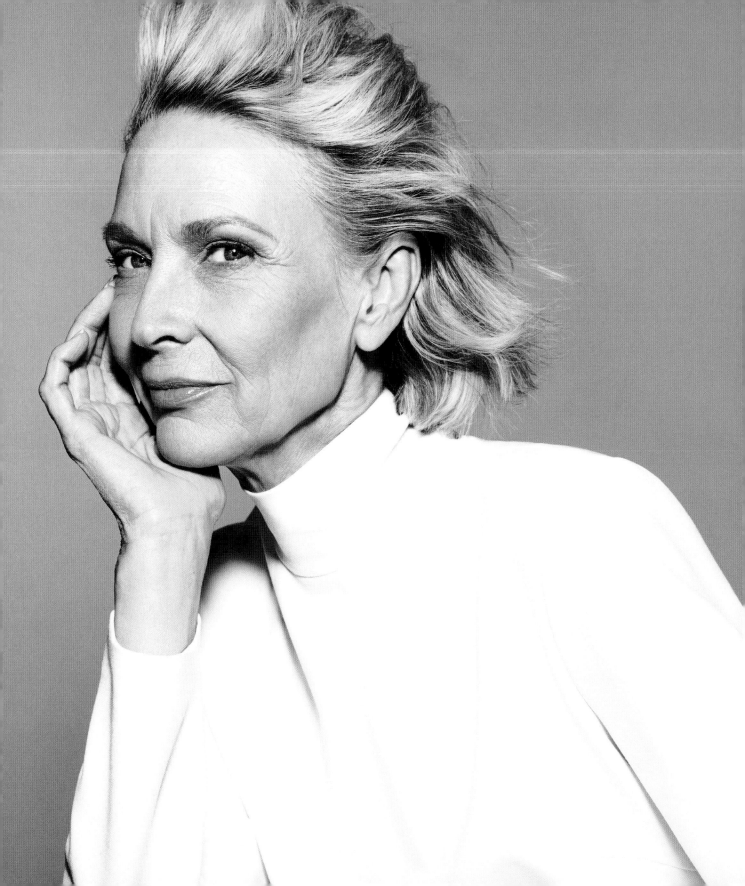

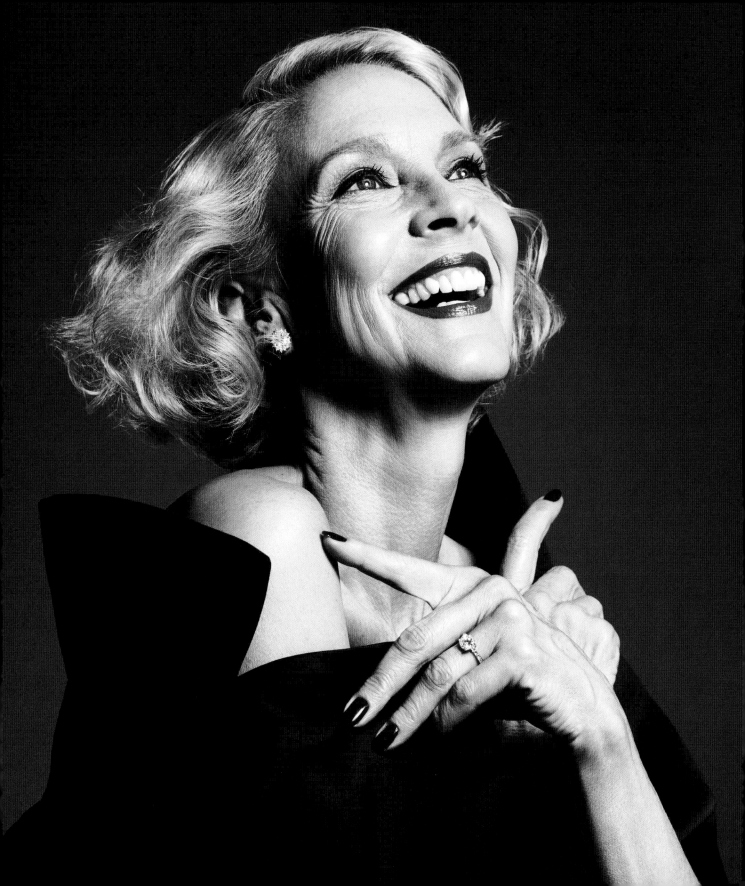

GALA LOOK

Because Karen will be wearing a black silk gown, I wanted her eye makeup to have some color. I chose a green-turquoise medium-matte eye shadow to really take Karen's beautiful eyes to another level. Medium-matte shadow reflects a little bit of light without too much of a shimmer effect—perfect for evening.

When using a dark eye shadow with lots of pigment, tap the brush on the box so the excess falls off and doesn't land on your cheeks. If that happens, wipe it off with a sponge moistened with a bit of foundation. This is a trick that makeup artists use.

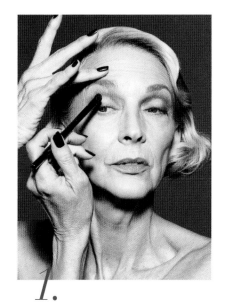

1.

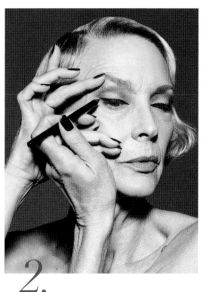

2.

1. Using your eye shadow brush, apply the shadow on the lash line and on the crease. Blend well with a blending brush.

2. Black waterproof eyeliner pencil creates the volume and drama needed for a big gala evening look. When lining the eyes, gently pull the skin taut to give yourself a straight canvas for smoother and easier application. Apply the liner to the waterline as well for a bolder finish. You can also squeeze your eyes shut after applying the pencil eyeliner on your waterline to get the color on the upper eye waterline—this is called tightlines. It makes your lashes look thicker! Waterproof liners dry quickly, so have a cotton swab handy in case you make a mistake.

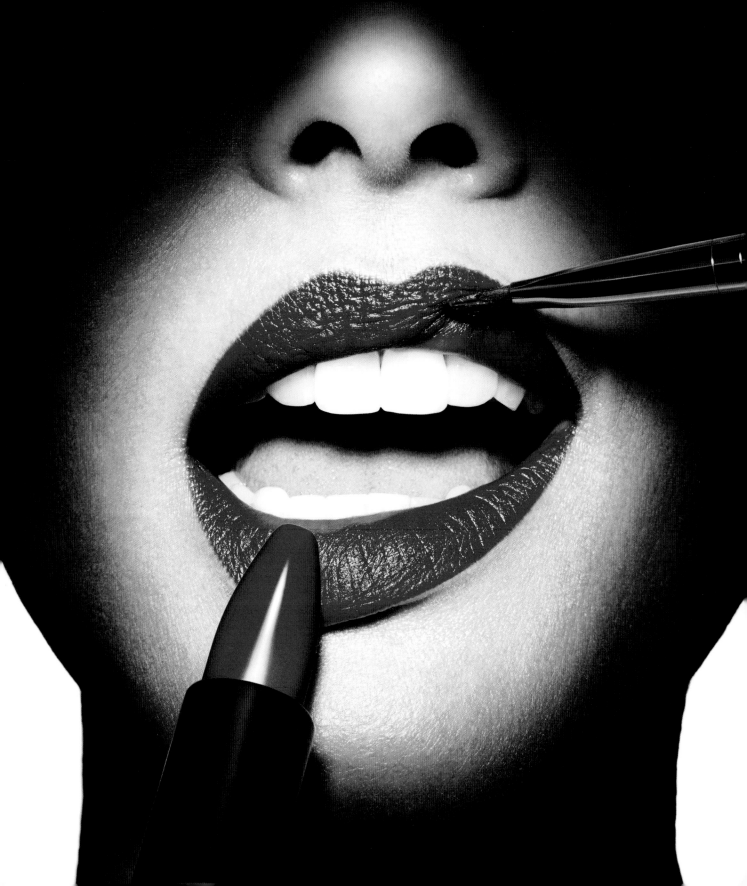

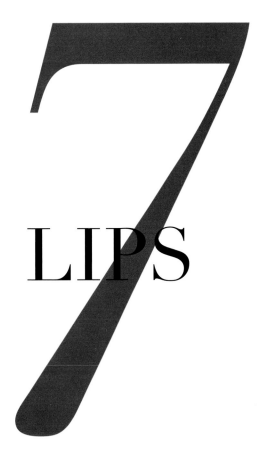

7

LIPS

The most-sold makeup product has always been lipstick, and that is not a surprise, because it is the fastest way to change your look. For mature women, lipstick—along with blush and mascara—is one of the easiest ways to acquire instant polish.

CHOOSING A LIPSTICK COLOR

The first thing to consider when choosing a new lipstick is the color. Your skin tone plays a big part in this. Below is a simple list that will help you make your decision.

Fair

- Even if you have blue undertones to your lips, pink—from light rose to raspberry to bright fuchsia—always looks great.

- Warm shades of red look fantastic, and I love bright orange-red lips on very light skin, which reminds me of 1950s classic Hollywood style. You can never go wrong with red lips. I also don't believe that red lipstick makes you look old. Absolutely not! It is the classiest makeup look ever.

- If you like nude colors, use muted rose, light peach, and coral.

- **Avoid:** All nudes that are gray and light, which will wash out your lips and make your teeth look yellow. Brown shades make your lips look smaller and age your face.

Tan

- Deep rose, mauve, raspberry, reddish brown, and burgundy always work.

- For more color, choose hot pink, fuchsia, magenta, purple, and cool reds.

- **Avoid:** Corals and orange-reds don't look good on skin that has yellow undertones. Nudes will totally wash out your lips.

Dark to ebony

- Deep brown, purple, and cool bluish reds always look fantastic on dark skin.

- Bright orange-reds and gold look amazing for evening.

- **Avoid:** Colors that are too light will make your lips look ashy.

CHOOSING A LIPSTICK TEXTURE

- For a natural result, choose a moisturizing lipstick that is not too glossy but still reflects light so the lips always look fresh. Use a lip primer under the lipstick so it stays well.

- Choose creamy formulas that have solid pigmentation and moisturizing ingredients (for example, shea butter).

- Choose a lip pencil that complements your lipstick color to line your lips. This will give you a sharp but natural boundary for the field of color.

- If you are not a lipstick woman, you can use a tinted lip balm, which will give you just a hint of color.

- **Avoid:** Long-lasting matte lipsticks always end up looking way too dry. Lip glosses are not a good choice, either, because they feather right away into the fine lines around the lips.

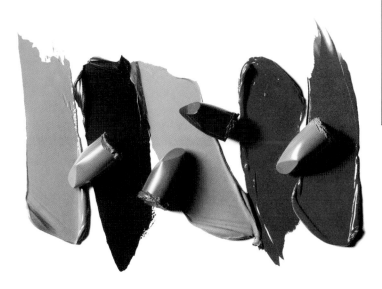

TO MAKE YOUR LIPSTICK LAST LONGER

1. Exfoliate your lips.
2. Use lip balm.
3. Use lip primer around and on the lips.
4. Line your lips with pencil.
5. Color in your lips with lip liner.
6. Apply lipstick on top of your lined lips.

TO MAKE YOUR LIPS LOOK FULLER

Your lips get thinner as you get older, but you can make them look fuller by outlining the lips just a few millimeters outside your natural lip line, especially in the corners.

If you wear a neutral lipstick, use a lip liner half a shade darker to instantly create a lip lift. Make sure the result looks natural: don't draw a line that's too thick.

APPLYING LIPSTICK

1. Your lips should always be moisturized before you apply lipstick. If they're dry, exfoliate them as well as the skin around your lips with a face scrub and warm water. Apply lip balm right afterward. Let it absorb into the skin for a few minutes. Then smooth a little bit of foundation on your lips to cover up your natural undertone. This will give you a neutral canvas on which to apply your color, allowing its full power to come through.

2. Line your lips with lip liner. This will build a "wall" around the lips: its waxy ingredients will encourage the lipstick to stay inside its boundaries.

3. Color in your lips with the lip liner.

4. Apply lipstick straight from the tube over your lips, either without lining them first or after you've lined them.

5. You can also use a lip brush to apply the lipstick.

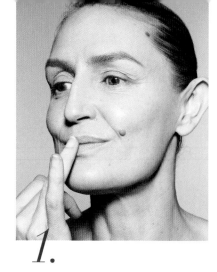

1.

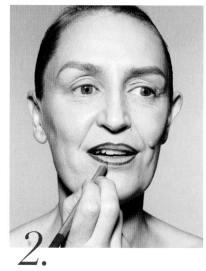

2.

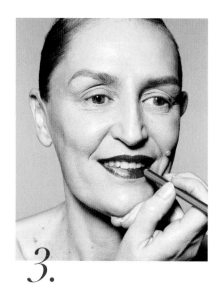

3.

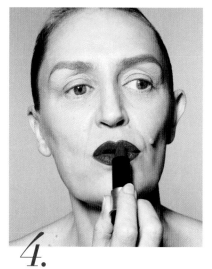

4.

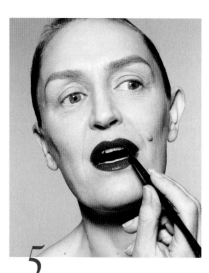

5.

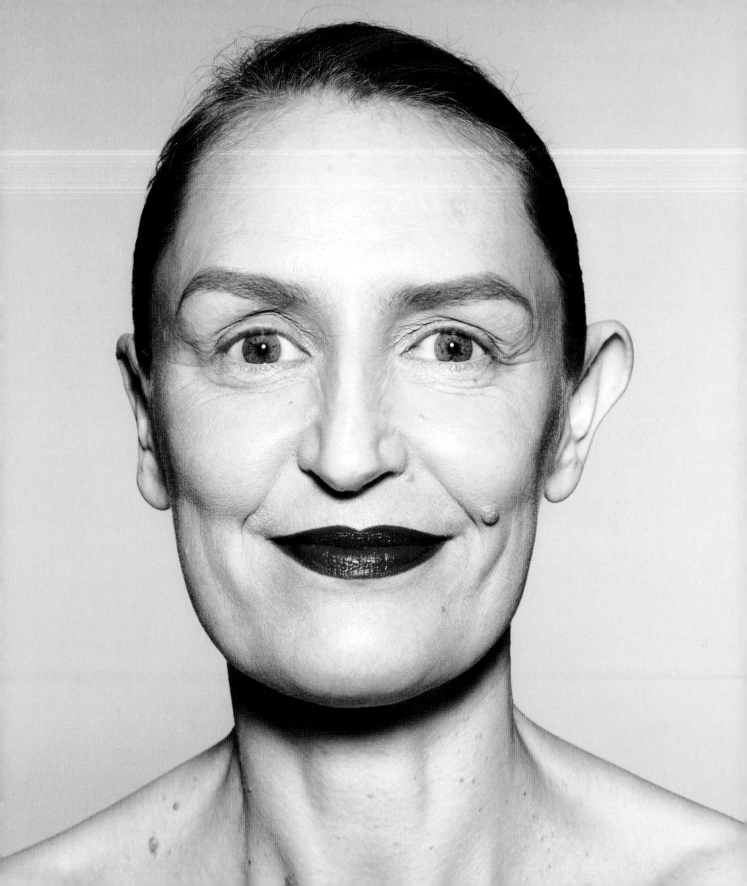

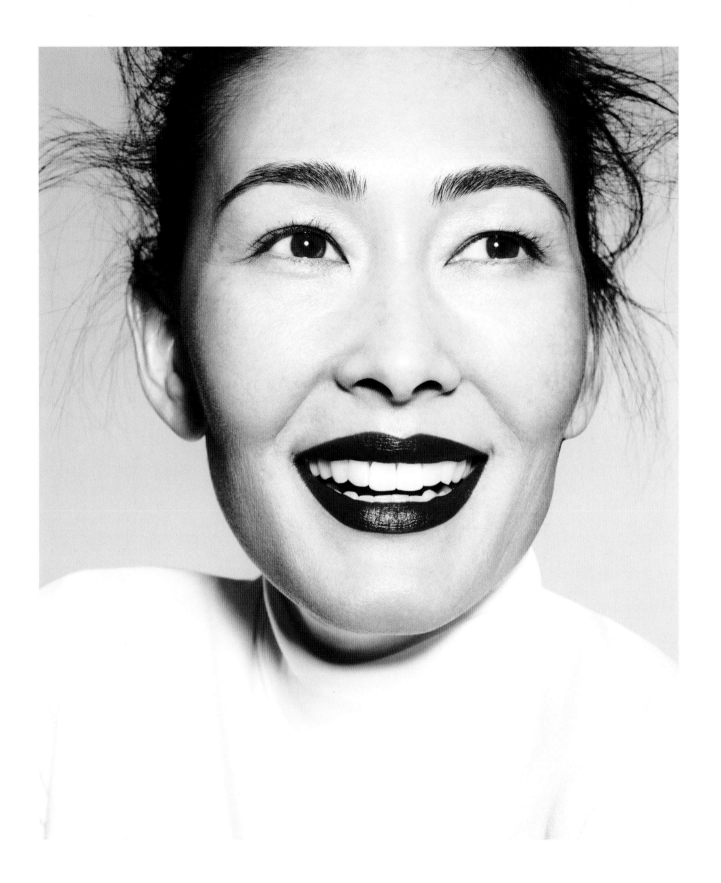

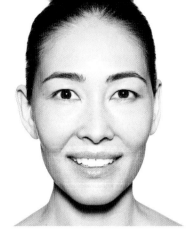

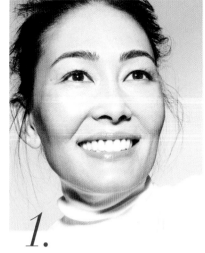

1.

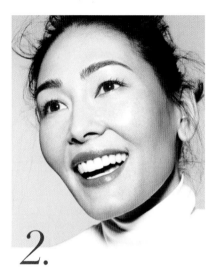

2.

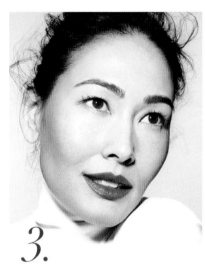

3.

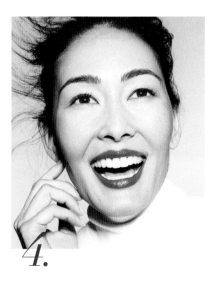

4.

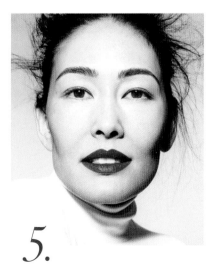

5.

CHANGE IT UP!

A simple change of lipstick color will completely transform your look.

1. Use a light peach nude sheer lipstick for a neutral and natural look that's great for everyday wear.

2. Apply a fresh pink sheer lipstick for versatility year-round.

3. Choose a color that's a bit deeper, such as this coral sheer lipstick, to brighten the face. This is a good option for the spring and summer.

4. Use an orange-red sheer lipstick if you want a bold spring and summer color.

5. For the classiest effect, one that always looks fantastic with minimal eye makeup, go with a red creamy semimatte lipstick.

To create a vampy, dramatic look for fall and winter evenings, wear a dark creamy semimatte lipstick (far left).

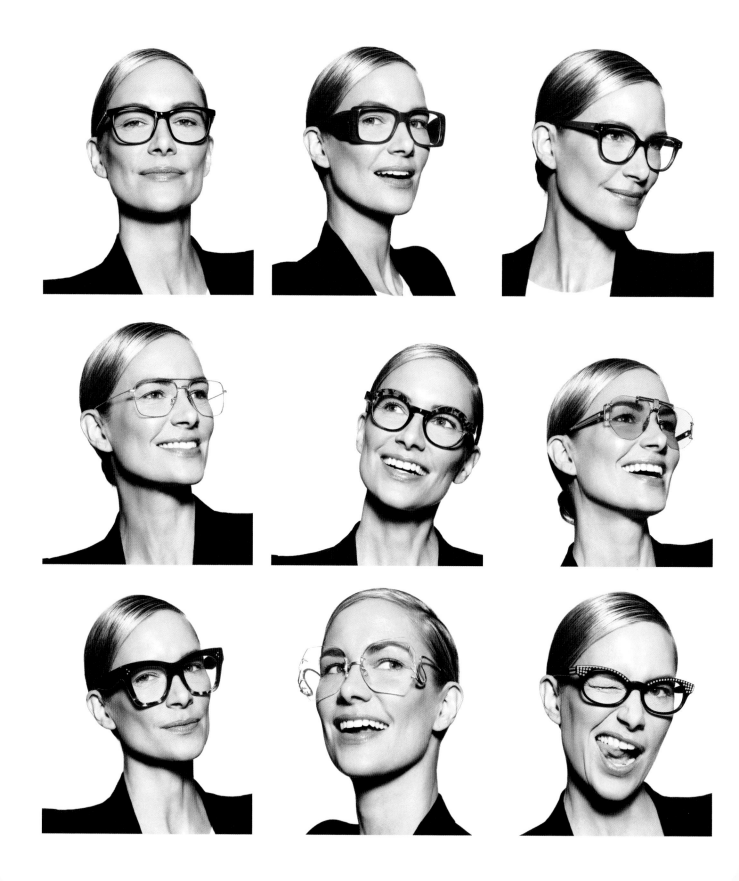

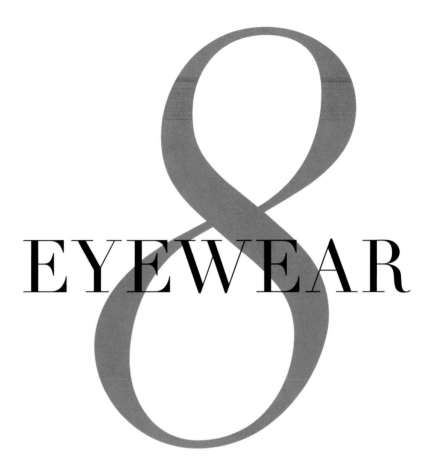

EYEWEAR

Eyewear is a fashion accessory that can uplift, upgrade, and modernize your look—if you choose the perfect frames. I interviewed Susan Sykes, who owns Eyes on Main in Santa Monica, California, and has been choosing frames for her clients for more than forty years.

What are the main factors to consider when choosing eyewear for a customer?

First and foremost are size and fit. The way a frame sits on the nose is extremely important for overall comfort. Size is critical, too. You want to have a good balance and have your eyes be fairly centered in the frame.

Styles, shapes, and colors are limitless, and it really depends on the client's personality, profession, budget, and lifestyle.

These days eyeglasses are not only necessary for some but also one of the most noticeable and important accessories you can own. Multiple looks can be achieved with various frames, so create a collection!

Does the prescription make any difference when choosing the frames?

Size and fit requirements can change with certain prescriptions. Large frames, for example, can have a direct impact on the thickness and weight of the final product. Some prescriptions can also have a negative impact on aesthetics. A good optician will direct you to a frame that can address your prescription and style requirements.

Can you wear metal frames if you have a nickel allergy?

Today's frames are made from many different materials, ranging from acetate to pure titanium, precious metals, and even carbon fiber. Certain metals can cause adverse reactions in some people—nickel is probably the biggest culprit. Metal frames, adjusted properly, should not come into contact with the skin.

How can you keep your eyewear in the best possible condition year after year?

Although most people replace their glasses around every two years, you can increase their longevity by taking care of them. Having them checked and adjusted periodically by a professional is key. Cleaning them with an optician-approved solution will help. Also, storing them in a case when not in use gives them extra life. Always remember to take your glasses off with both hands.

Once you have picked out your frames, it's time to think about the best makeup choices to go with your new eyewear.

FOUNDATION AND FRAMES

Lots of women who wear foundation (or tinted moisturizer or just concealer alone) have a persistent problem: how to keep their eyeglasses from leaving marks on the nose. Follow the steps below to prevent this.

1. On clean skin, apply eyelid primer to both sides of the nose. Use a brush, a sponge, or your finger to tap on your concealer or foundation. Then powder the area. This will also help the foundation last longer.

2. Don't use too much foundation. Just the lightest covering will give you beautiful, natural, light-reflecting dewy skin. And where there isn't a lot of foundation, not a lot will come off. So use a light hydrating foundation and blend it well.

3. To help your eyelids blend well with the rest of your skin, remember to cover them with foundation so any discoloration will be camouflaged.

CONCEALER

Because eyeglass frames might create shadows around the eyes, I always recommend using concealer to lighten and lift the eye area, especially in the inner corners, where the deepest shadows lie. I am not a big fan of light-reflecting pencils, because they can bring out the fine lines around your eyes. Stick with concealer.

EYEBROWS

Some eyeglass frames cover your brows completely, so you don't really need to fill in your brows. Be aware that lenses for farsighted people magnify the eyes and can show all the fine hairs under your brows. If the frames you wear show your brows, you can fill them in or just leave them looking natural. It depends on your personal style.

TIPS FOR NEARSIGHTED PEOPLE

- Your lenses can make your eyes look smaller. Avoid too-dark eye shadow and dark eyeliner, especially on the waterline, which can make your eyes look even smaller.

- Use nude eye shadow on the lids, medium-dark shadow (depending on your skin color) into the crease and lash line, and white or nude pencil liner on the waterline.

- Curl your lashes if needed and apply black mascara to open up your eyes. Waterproof mascara helps your lashes stay curled longer.

- You can also use just a thin colorful pencil liner only on your upper lash line. This brings out your eyes beautifully.

TIPS FOR FARSIGHTED PEOPLE

- Your lenses can make your eyes look bigger—but fortunately, making the eyes look smaller is easy. Use a dark pencil liner (black, dark brown, dark gray, navy blue, or dark, dark green) on the upper lash line and waterline. On the bottom waterline, use a chocolate-brown waterproof pencil liner and a black pencil liner for a dramatic look.

- Always use a waterproof eye pencil so it will stay on your eyes the whole day. Right after you have applied the pencil to the lash line, smudge it a bit so it looks softer through the lenses.

- You can also use any color matte eye shadow that goes with your skin tone on the entire lid up to the socket as well as on the bottom lash line.

- Avoid shimmery, glittery shadows because they will show the fine lines on your lids.

EYE SHADOW

Use matte eye shadow during the daytime. A slightly more light-reflecting shadow can be used for the evening.

I recommend that you apply eyelid primer, foundation, and powder to prevent your shadow and liner from creasing.

Don't use cream shadows—they will crease, even though they're not supposed to. Stick with the powdered format.

MASCARA

Use waterproof mascara. It won't smudge on your lenses, and if your eyes are watery, it won't run.

FALSE EYELASHES

The only false eyelashes I recommend are individual lashes in the shortest possible length. If you don't wear those, skip them altogether. They will touch your glasses and make you feel uncomfortable. If you do wear them, make sure to only put a small amount of clear eyelash glue on the base of the false lash, wait twenty seconds for it to get tacky, then carefully apply with tweezers as close to the lash line as possible.

FRAMES AND MAKEUP STYLES

Following are six different frame styles with makeup and hair looks to match.

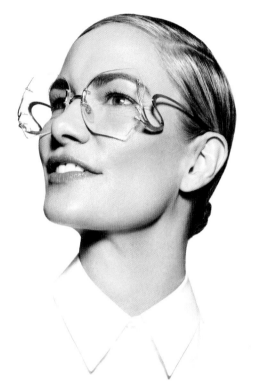

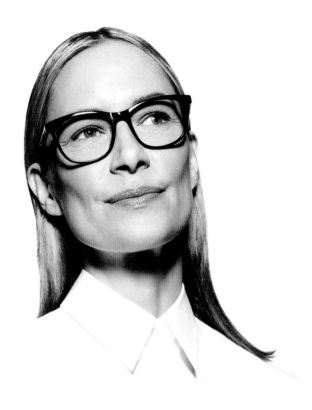

Large frameless lenses

This style creates lots of space around the eyes, and because the design is bold, you'll want to leave your eye makeup very open and natural. Apply only warm beige matte eye shadow and black mascara, and fill your brows in slightly to provide a natural frame for the eyes. Choose a fresh peach-coral lipstick to complement the natural eye makeup, and finish with a touch of blush.

Black acrylic frames

This type of frame calls for the same makeup look as the frameless style—open and natural. You can see how much the frames change Allison's face just by covering her eyebrows.

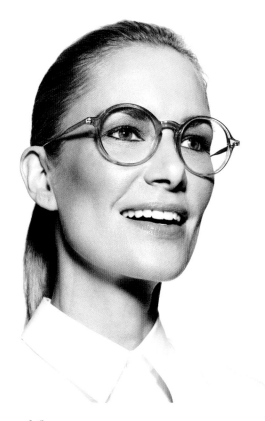

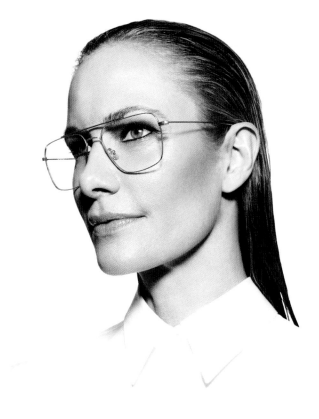

Round frames

Because lenses to correct farsightedness make the eyes look bigger, use a chocolate-brown waterproof eye pencil on the waterlines and the upper lash line to minimize the eyes. Apply a warm matte eye shadow—the same color as the frames—to create a monochrome look. Choose a deep peach blush that will go hand in hand with a similar color lipstick.

Metallic silver frames

For an evening occasion, use a black pencil liner on the upper and lower waterlines and upper lash line to accentuate the eyes. Because the frames are very modern and light and create lots of space around the eyes, you will want to keep the look smoky. To keep the effect ultramodern and cool, don't put anything on your lips except lip balm, and use a light matte bronzer on your cheeks.

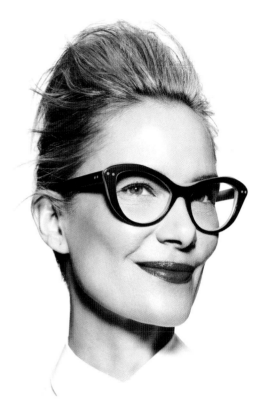

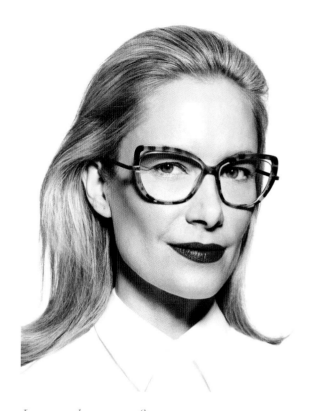

Turquoise-accented cat-eye frames

Apply turquoise pencil liner to the upper lash line. Curl your lashes, then apply separating mascara to bring out the eyes and keep the emphasis on the upper lids. Use a nude eyeliner on the waterlines. To bring more attitude, line and fill the lips in bright coral.

Leopard cat-eye frames

When the frames are this big and incorporate multiple colors or prints, it is better to leave the eye makeup minimal but make the lips stand out. Use a very thin black pencil liner on the upper lash line and a white pencil liner on the lower waterline to open up the eyes. Coordinate the makeup color with the frames: a creamy, dark reddish-brown lipstick goes hand in hand with the brown-and-tan pattern, creating a bold look.

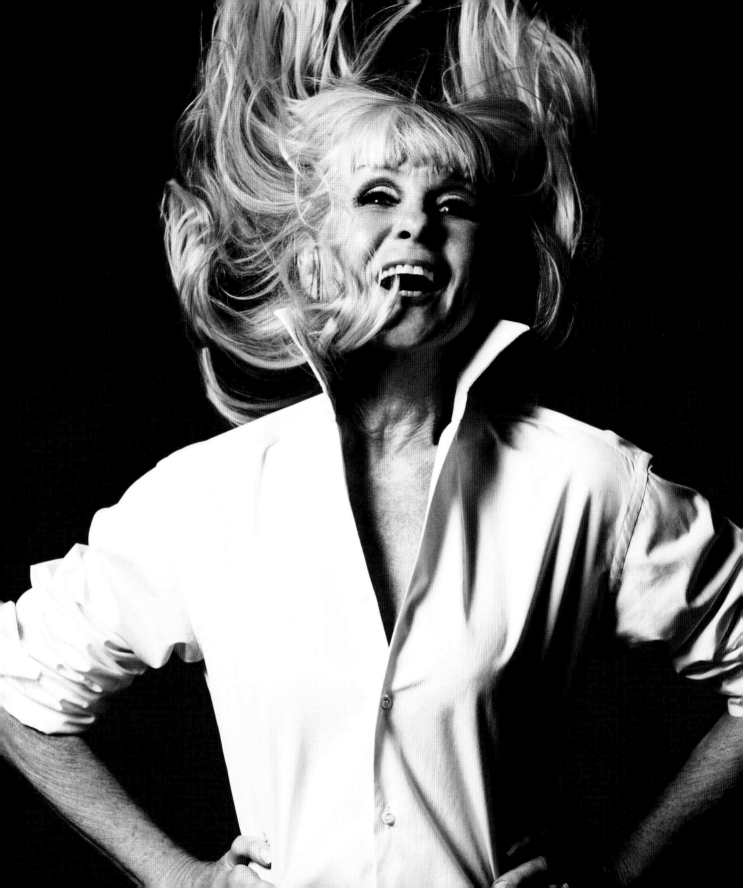

BEAUTY *in* ACTION

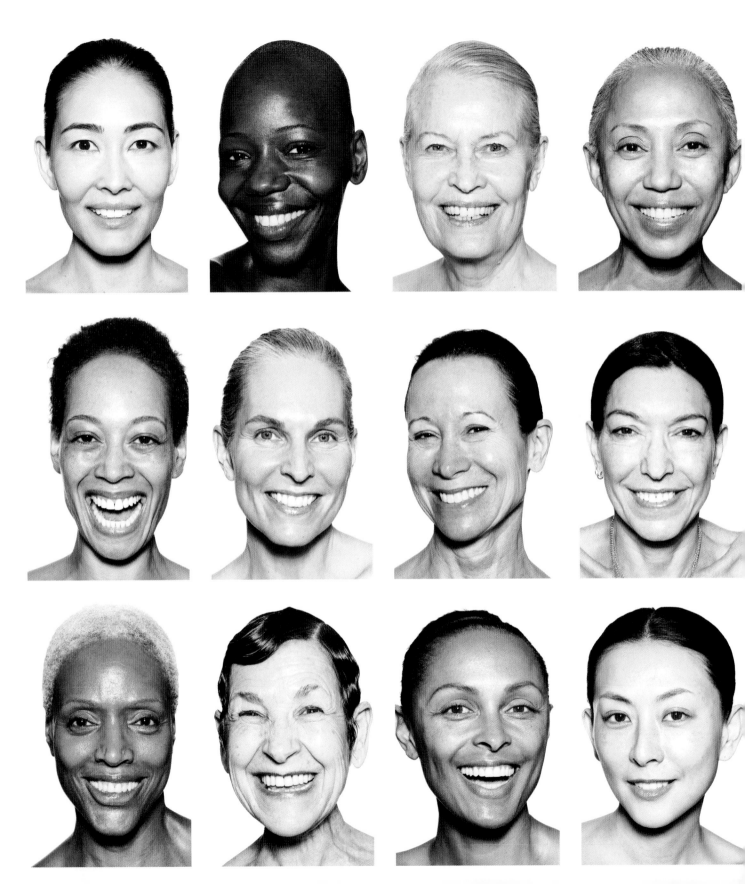

MAKEOVERS

For this part, I chose sixteen different women of various races, sizes, and ages (all 40 and older, of course). Each woman wears two different looks—one for daytime and one for evening—based on her personality and lifestyle.

Before any makeup was applied, each model was treated to my mini facial, which includes

- double-cleansing with cleansing milk,

- spritzing with toner,

- an application of serum,

- an eye cream or eye mask, and

- a generous dollop of hydrating deep-moisturizing face cream, which I massaged into the skin and tapped with my fingers into the face and neck.

Prior to these makeovers, we also applied foundation, concealer, color corrector, powder, and often lip, eye, or face primer. For instructions on applying foundation, please see chapter 3.

Get inspired and enjoy!

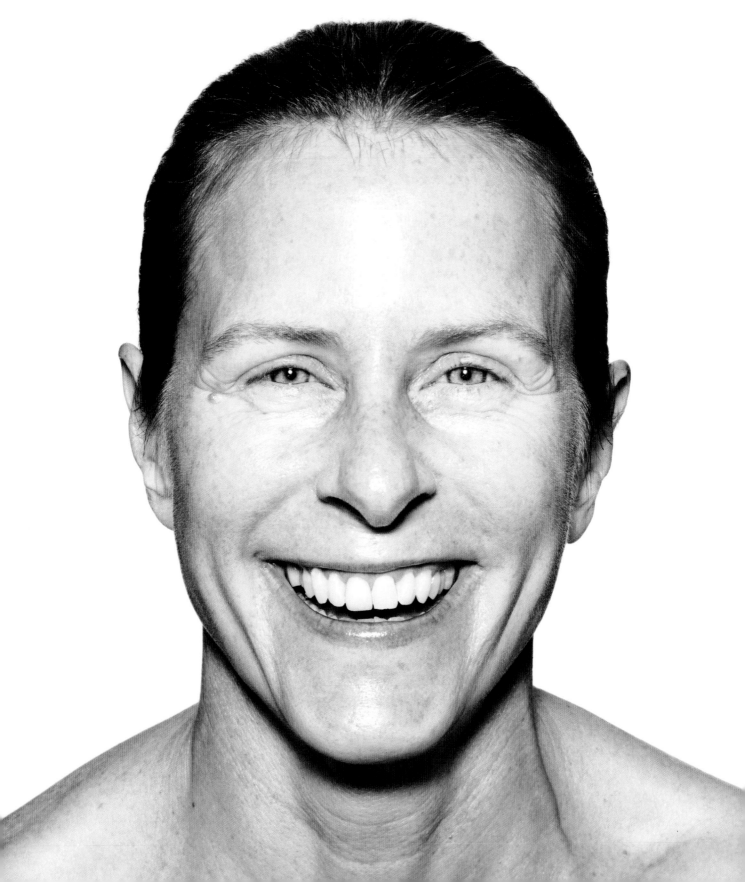

MODERN GRUNGE
TERESA

Teresa, 55, is a New York–based film/photo producer, and because of her busy schedule, she prefers a quick application of makeup that will last all day and give her a natural, dewy glow.

Are there any beauty tips or tricks your family members passed on to you that you still use?

Without question, my mother insisted that I wash my face and brush my teeth before bed. I never leave the house without doing both. Also, my sister Lynn told me early on that "a little goes a long way." If you don't want to wear full makeup, just color your lips.

How has the meaning of beauty changed for you through the years?

Georgia O'Keeffe was the epitome of beauty: she never altered her face. The stories that lived in each deep line of her face, the history—I see such beauty in that. I will always see beauty there. Sometimes it's what you don't do that creates beauty, and as I age, I see that embracing our years is what constitutes true beauty.

What are your daily beauty routines?

I am into organic, clean, and green products. I use face and body oils and organic sunblock.

Do you have any beauty wisdom for the next generation?

Protect your skin from the sun. Buy sunscreen that doesn't contain toxic chemicals such as oxybenzone, avobenzone, octisalate, octocrylene, homosalate, and octinoxate. Always consider what you're doing to the vessel that is your body. Most important, be happy, love, and laugh a lot . . . life is so short!

What makes you feel beautiful?

Lingerie! I wear lingerie for myself. The way it makes me feel is beautiful. Nobody knows I'm wearing it but me. And when I let someone else see it, all the better!

What is your motto for life?

The biggest risk in life is not risking anything. Let fear be your biggest inspiration.

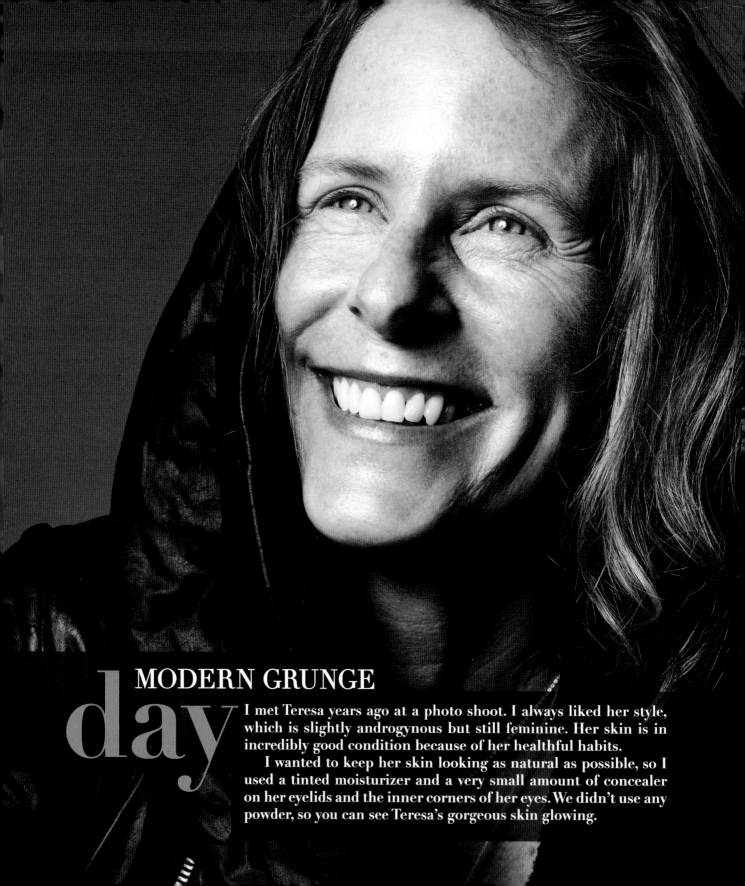

MODERN GRUNGE

day

I met Teresa years ago at a photo shoot. I always liked her style, which is slightly androgynous but still feminine. Her skin is in incredibly good condition because of her healthful habits.

I wanted to keep her skin looking as natural as possible, so I used a tinted moisturizer and a very small amount of concealer on her eyelids and the inner corners of her eyes. We didn't use any powder, so you can see Teresa's gorgeous skin glowing.

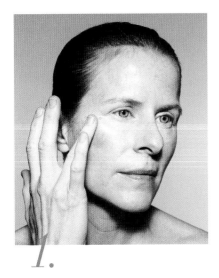

1.

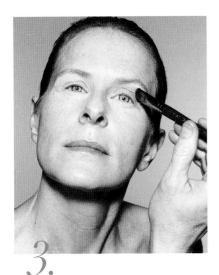

3.

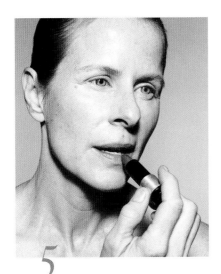

5.

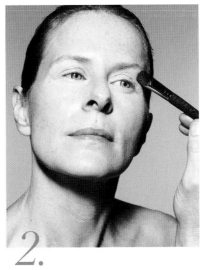

2.

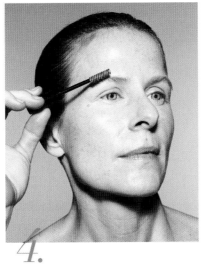

4.

1. After applying the base products, Teresa tapped cream blush on her cheeks with her fingers. I wanted to keep her makeup tones in the earthy color family so all the colors would blend well together.

2. A light matte eye shadow was applied all over her lids up to the brow bone with a blending brush (#8 on page 25). This was applied on top of the tinted moisturizer, so the shadow works as a powder and opens up her eyes at the same time. I didn't use mascara because I wanted her eyes to look as natural as possible.

3. Then Teresa applied a slightly darker shadow in the crease of her eyelid.

4. She brushed her brows with brow gel to give them some shine and to make sure they stayed in place during the day.

5. Teresa then applied lip balm followed by lipstick in a warm tone straight from the tube.

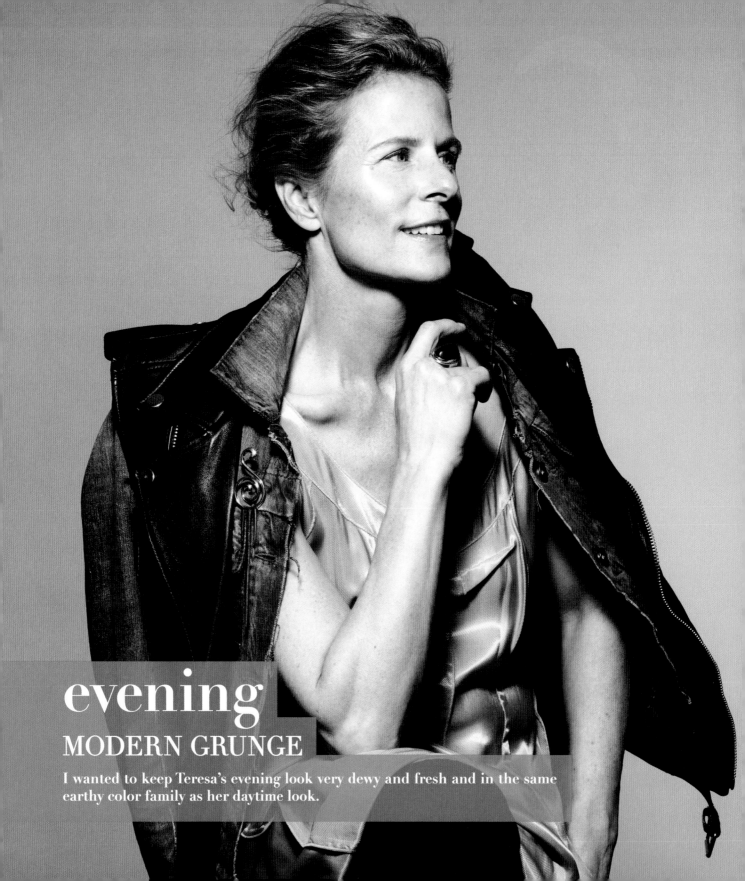

evening
MODERN GRUNGE

I wanted to keep Teresa's evening look very dewy and fresh and in the same earthy color family as her daytime look.

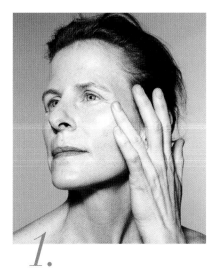

1.

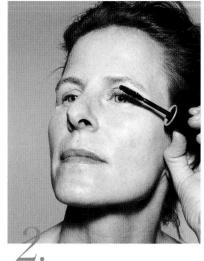

2.

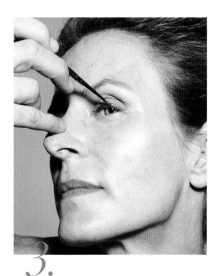

3.

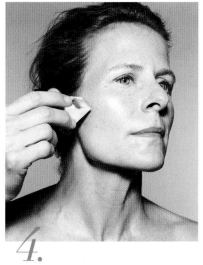

4.

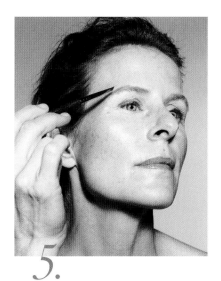

5.

1. After applying tinted moisturizer, Teresa tapped golden highlighter on her cheeks to bring out her high cheekbones.

2. After curling her lashes, she applied black mascara.

3. Here she applied light-reflecting bronze waterproof liner with an eyeliner brush (#11 on page 25). She didn't use it on the inner corners of the eyes, just on the lash line.

4. Teresa applied cream bronzer below the highlighter to give warmth to the face.

5. She used a warm taupe to fill in the eyebrows with a brow brush (#10). Teresa also applied brow gel to keep the hairs in place.

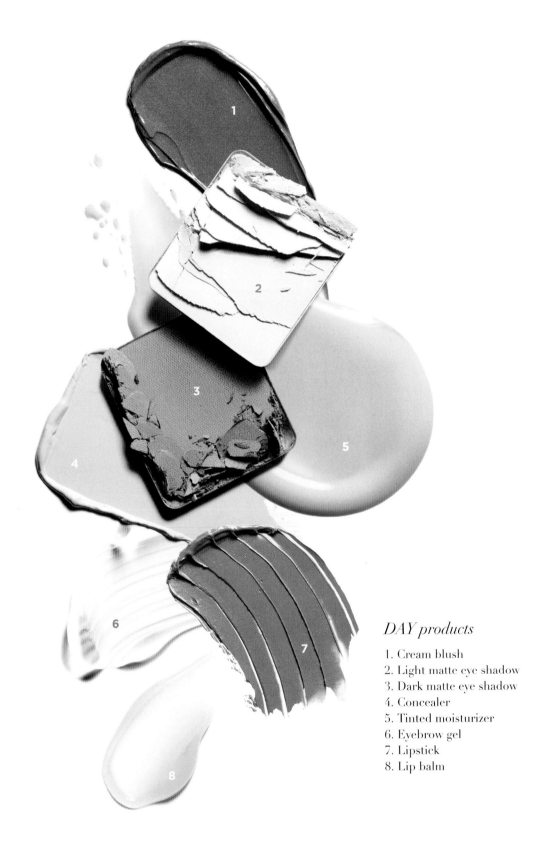

DAY products

1. Cream blush
2. Light matte eye shadow
3. Dark matte eye shadow
4. Concealer
5. Tinted moisturizer
6. Eyebrow gel
7. Lipstick
8. Lip balm

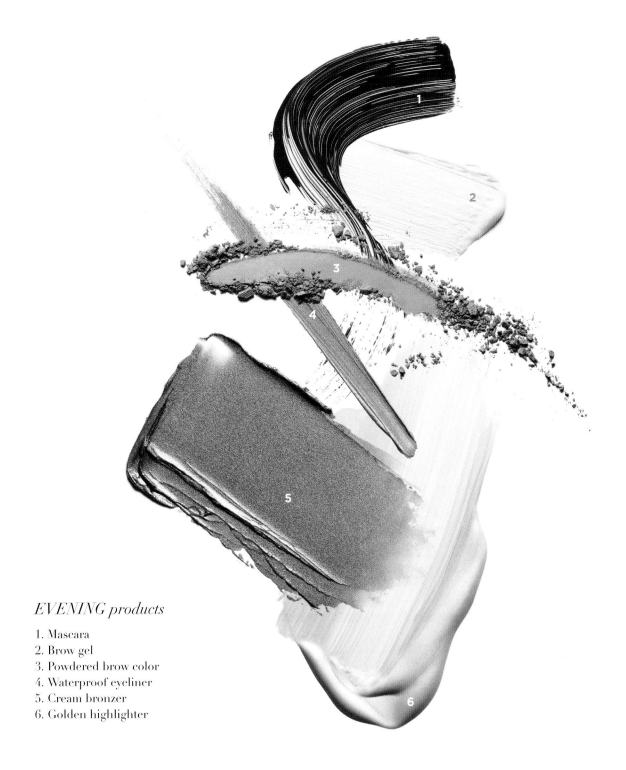

EVENING products

1. Mascara
2. Brow gel
3. Powdered brow color
4. Waterproof eyeliner
5. Cream bronzer
6. Golden highlighter

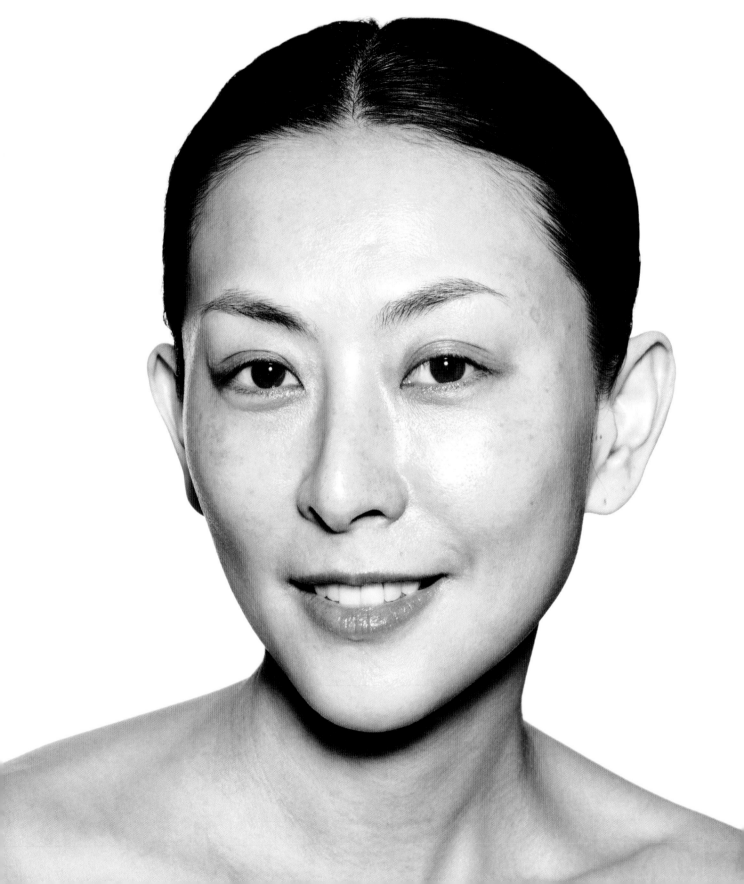

48 MINIMALIST TAMIYO

Japanese-born Tamiyo, 48, is a successful New York–based interior designer. Her simple style and beautiful skin inspired me to create these minimalist makeup looks that are wearable in any season—just choose the right foundation, blush, and lip color for your skin tone.

Are there any beauty tips or tricks your family members passed on to you that you still use?

Drink lots of water. Appreciate and respect other people: this helps maintain purity and a beautiful mind.

How has the meaning of beauty changed for you through the years?

Outer beauty doesn't last long, but inner beauty remains. I have regrets in my life and have made many mistakes, and those experiences have shaped me and helped make me beautiful. I have flaws, and those are beautiful.

What are your daily beauty routines?

I always eat until I am 80 percent full. I try to maintain great posture and attitude. I use toner twice a day after I wash my face, and I use sunscreen every single day, even when I stay indoors.

Do you have any beauty wisdom for the next generation?

Don't compare yourself to others. It will make you vain and insecure.

What does beauty mean to you?

Beauty means feeling comfortable in my own skin and appreciating imperfections.

What is your motto for life?

Life dies and rises like the moon.

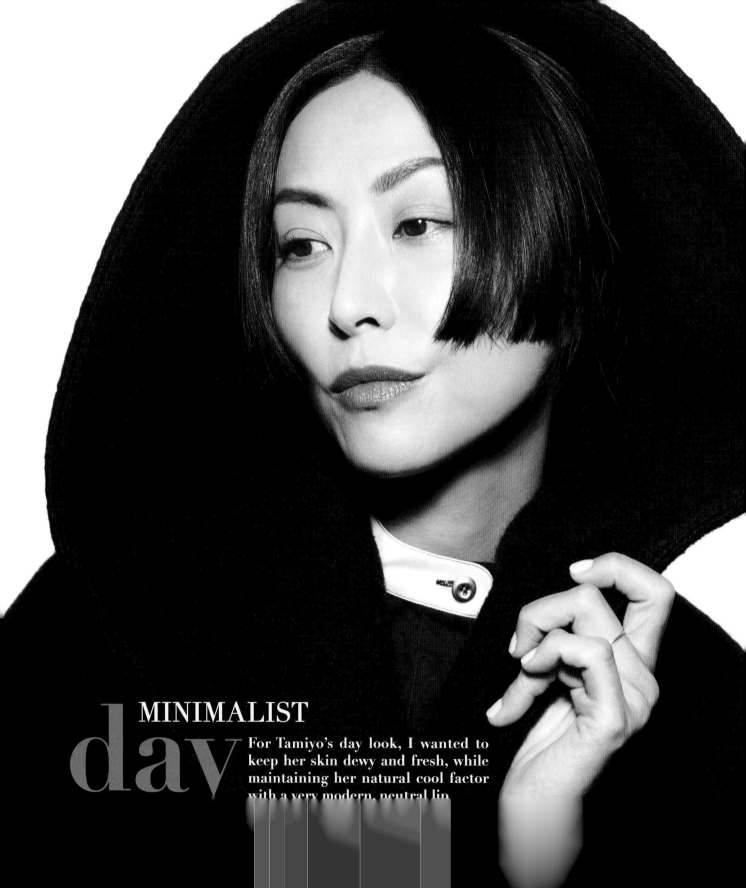

MINIMALIST
day

For Tamiyo's day look, I wanted to keep her skin dewy and fresh, while maintaining her natural cool factor with a very modern, neutral lip.

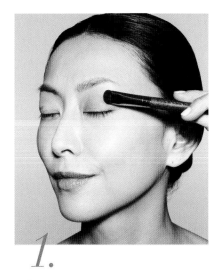

1.

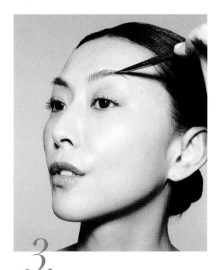

3.

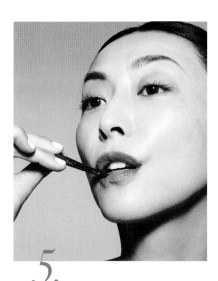

5.

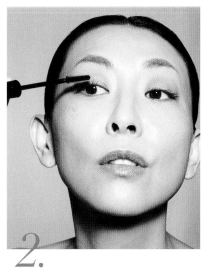

2.

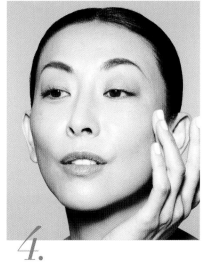

4.

1. A light beige matte eye shadow was applied to the whole eyelid up to the crease with a blending brush (#8 on page 25). This color is a tiny bit darker than Tamiyo's skin, so it gives a hint of definition to the eyes.

2. After curling her lashes, Tamiyo applied two coats of black waterproof mascara. Waterproof mascara helps your lashes stay curled longer.

3. Then she filled her brows with shadow using a brow brush (#10). Be light-handed, so the color blends and settles naturally. Afterward, she brushed her brows with gel to keep them in place.

4. Tamiyo applied a warm cream blush with her fingers to the apples of her cheeks. She tapped and blended well so it looks like she just blushed a little.

5. I chose a cool pink sheer lipstick that looks very natural on Tamiyo's lips. Even though the color is bright in the tube, it appears natural when applied with a light hand. You can apply the lipstick straight from the tube, tap it on with your fingers, or brush it on with a lip brush (#12).

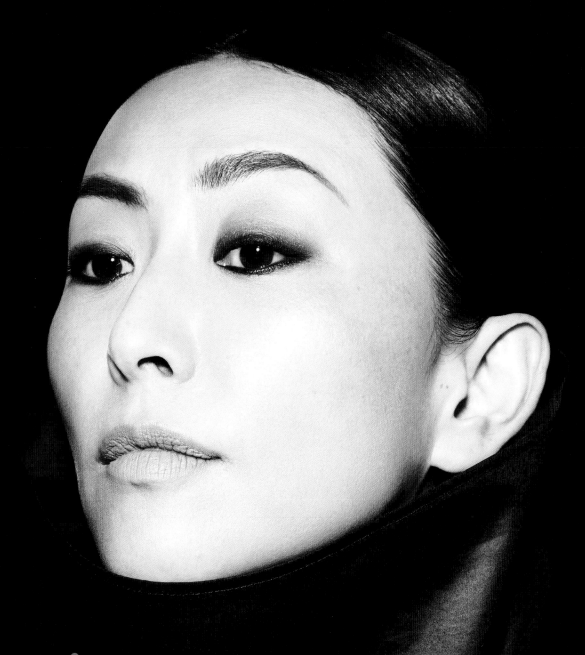

evening

MINIMALIST

Tamiyo's evening look is all about smoky eyes for a little edge. If eye pencil creases on your lids, use an eyelid primer before applying foundation and powder. That will guarantee staying power.

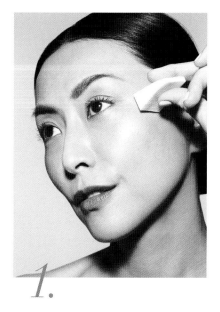

1.

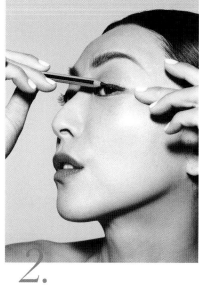

2.

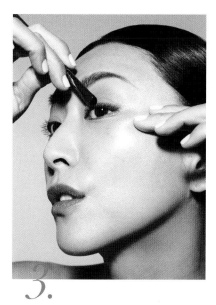

3.

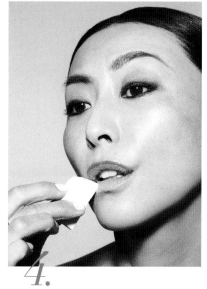

4.

1. Golden highlighter was applied on the cheeks to replace blush with the help of a latex-free triangle-shaped sponge, then blended well so the color melted into the skin and reflected subdued lighting beautifully.

2. Smoky eye makeup starts with a black eyeliner pencil. Tamiyo stretched her eye at the outer corner so she could easily draw the liner on the lash line. Then she blended with a small brush (#7 on page 25).

3. Lining Tamiyo's waterline really brought out her eyes and gave her makeup instant attitude. She also lined her bottom lash line, then blended it with the same brush she used in step 2.

4. Tamiyo applied foundation to her lips with a sponge to get very fashionable "foundation lips." They work well with smoky eyes in evening lighting.

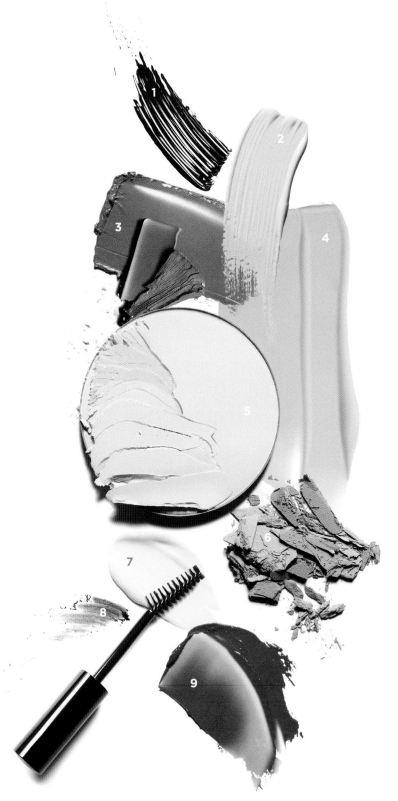

DAY products

1. Waterproof mascara
2. Concealer
3. Cream blush
4. Light hydrating foundation
5. Pressed powder
   (dusted on the lids and
   very lightly on the T-zone)
6. Matte eye shadow
7. Brow gel
8. Brow color
9. Sheer lipstick

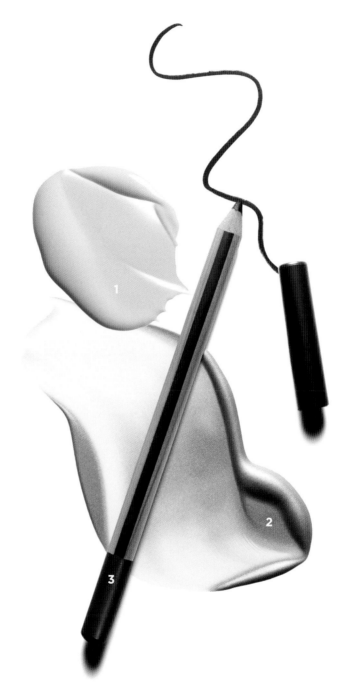

EVENING *products*

1. Foundation for the lips
2. Golden highlighter
3. Eye pencil

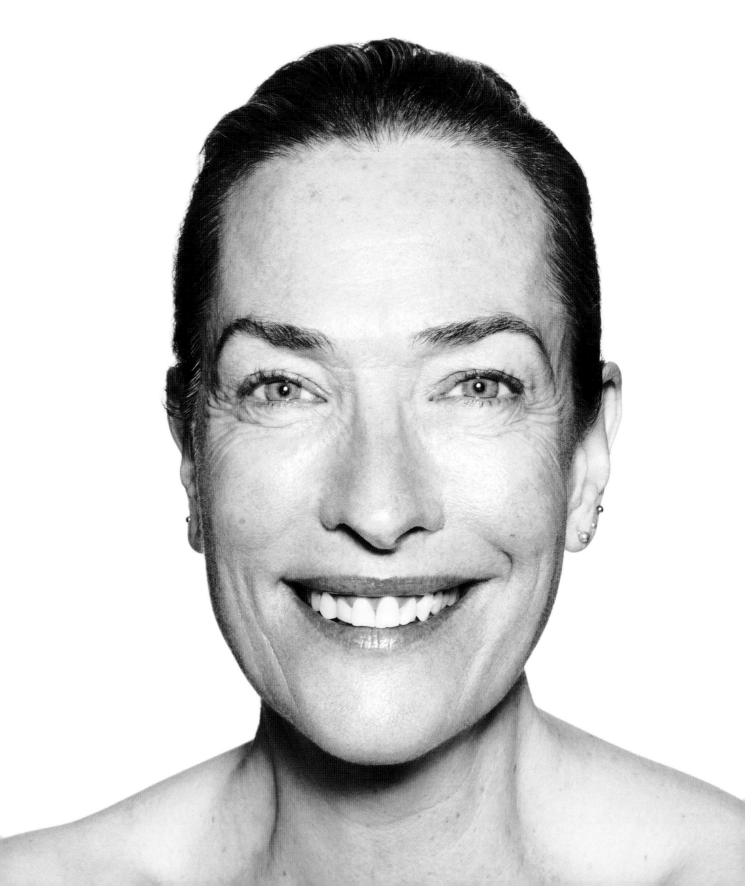

NATURAL BEAUTY
TATJANA

German-born Tatjana, 52, is a true natural beauty and one of the biggest supermodels of the 1980s and '90s. Her face has graced the covers of many international fashion magazines, and she has starred in many designers' advertising campaigns. Tatjana is also one of the all-time favorite models of Anna Wintour, Vogue's editor in chief. Today, Tatjana lives by the ocean in California and enjoys a very healthful lifestyle that includes organic food, skincare, and body care. She is also a big animal lover and takes care of two horses on her ranch.

Are there any beauty tips or tricks your family members passed on to you that you still use?

My grandmother always told me that you can find beauty aids in nature. For tired eyes, press them with chamomile tea bags (cold, of course). Use cucumber face masks, and put lemon juice in your hair in the summertime for natural highlights.

How has the meaning of beauty changed for you through the years?

True beauty is the whole person, from the inside out.

What are your daily beauty routines?

I cleanse first, then apply a face serum and moisturizer. It's very simple, really. Because I live in California, I use sunblock (SPF 30–50) daily, all year round.

Do you have any beauty wisdom for the next generation?

Take care of your skin, and it will take care of you.

What makes you feel beautiful?

Being happy and laughing makes me feel beautiful, especially when I'm around great friends, family, my pets, and nature.

What is your motto for life?

Feel gratitude and love.

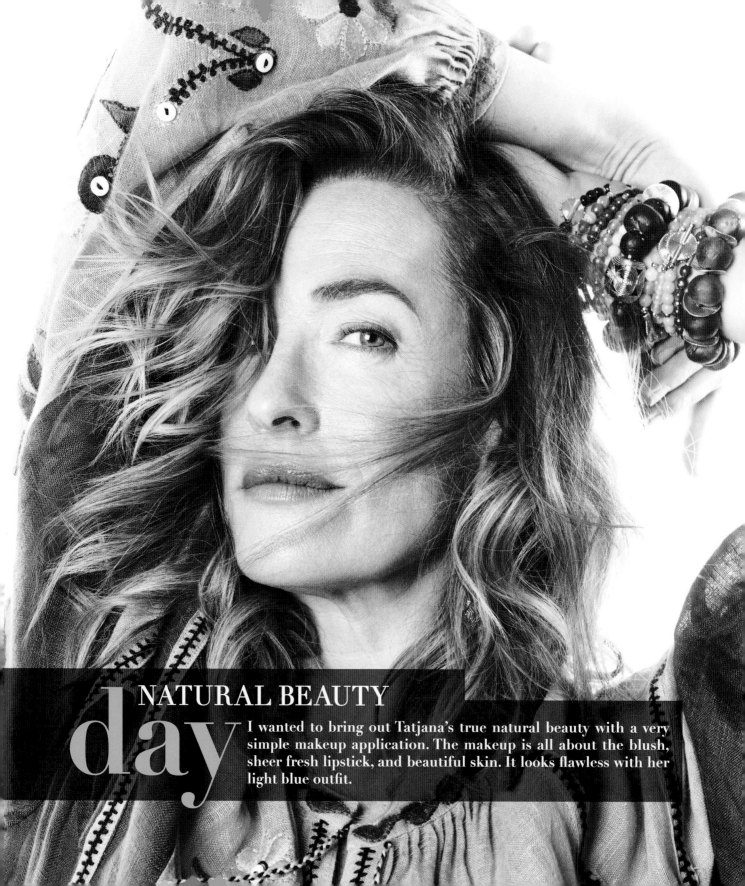

NATURAL BEAUTY

day

I wanted to bring out Tatjana's true natural beauty with a very simple makeup application. The makeup is all about the blush, sheer fresh lipstick, and beautiful skin. It looks flawless with her light blue outfit.

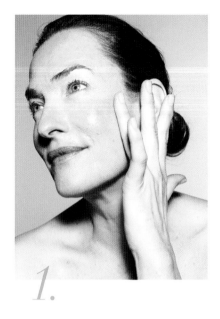

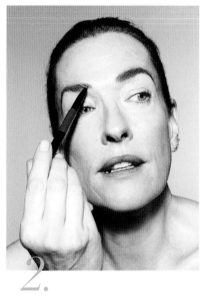

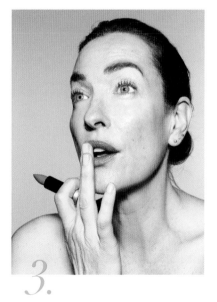

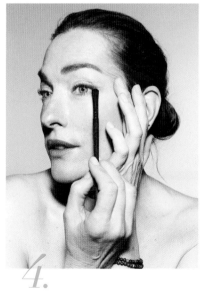

1. Sheer peach cream blush was applied with the fingers and blended on the apples of the cheeks to give a beautiful sheen and natural color.

2. Tatjana used a pencil to fill in her brows with a warm brown color, then brushed it through. She also curled her lashes and applied one coat of black mascara to open up her eyes.

3. She then applied peach sheer lipstick straight from the tube and evened out the color with her fingers.

4. To give more volume, Tatjana applied a brown matte eye shadow on the roots of the lashes with a small eye shadow brush (#7 on page 25).

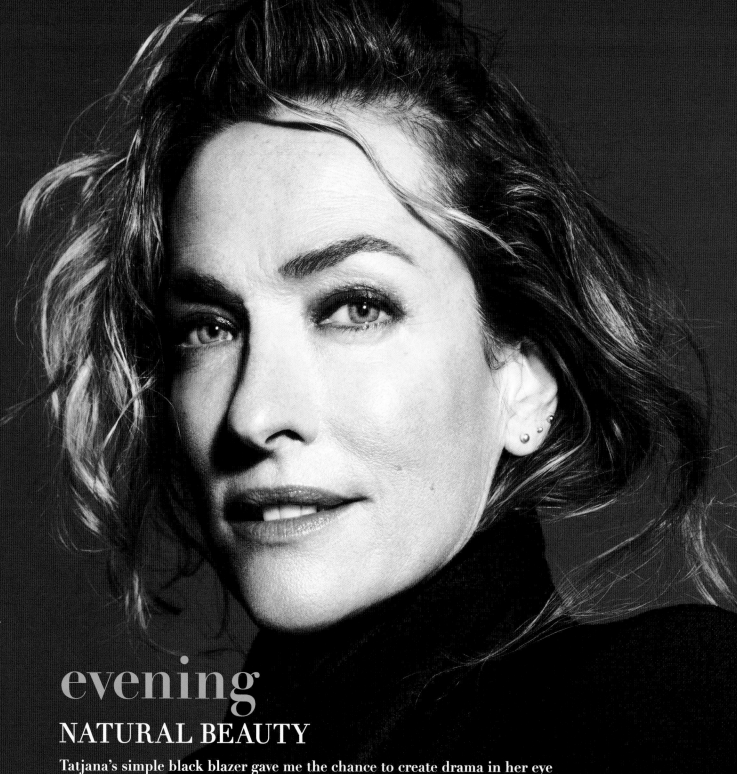

evening
NATURAL BEAUTY

Tatjana's simple black blazer gave me the chance to create drama in her eye makeup. I didn't use any lipstick, so the makeup looks modern. This look was applied on top of the day look.

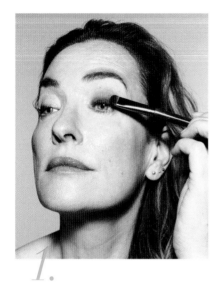

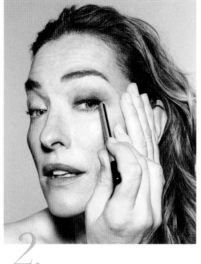

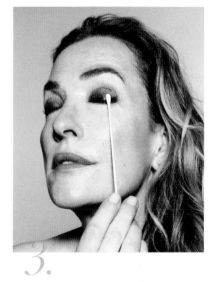

1. Tatjana applied blue matte eye shadow to the roots of her upper lash line with a small round brush (#7 on page 25). Then she blended it upward to create a color fade.

2. She applied black pencil liner to the roots of the lashes, then blended it with the brush.

3. Then, using a cotton swab, she applied a tiny bit of Elizabeth Arden's Eight Hour Cream Skin Protectant to her lids to bring on the shine. The shadow will crease on the lids, but it looks really cool in evening lighting.

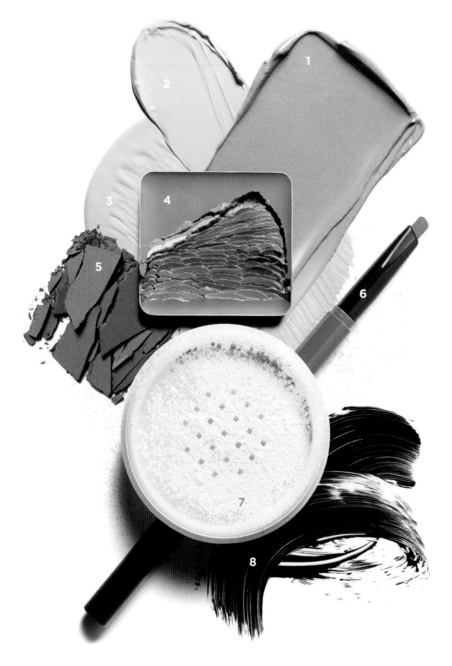

DAY products

1. Sheer lipstick
2. Concealer
3. Tinted moisturizer
4. Cream blush
5. Matte eye shadow
6. Brow pencil
7. Loose powder
8. Mascara

EVENING products

1. Matte eye shadow
2. Elizabeth Arden's Eight Hour
   Cream Skin Protectant
3. Eyeliner pencil

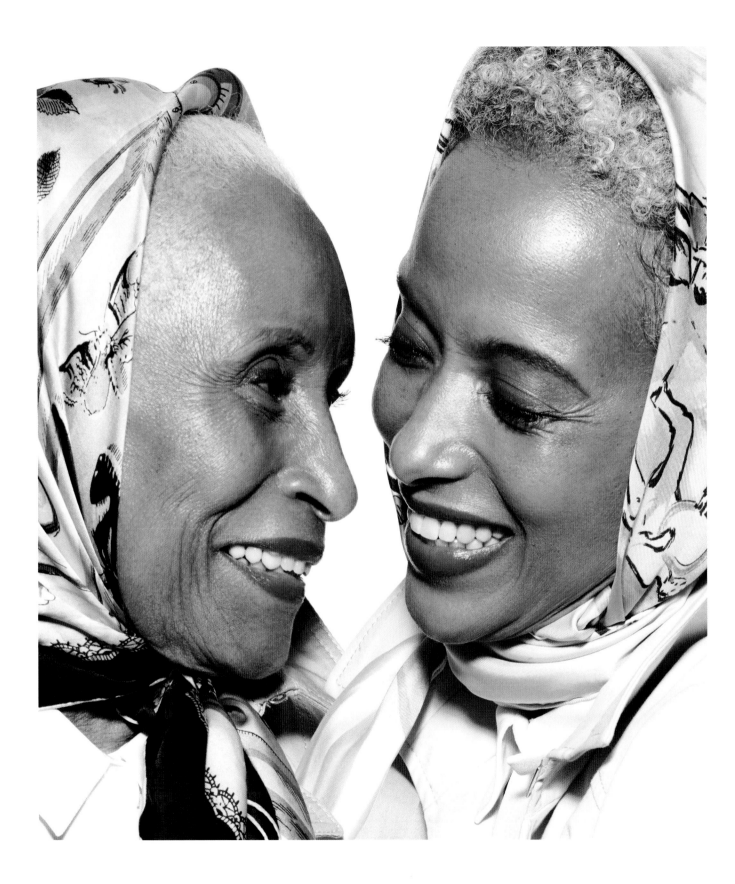

SPRING— DAUGHTER AND MOTHER

Spring is always a long-awaited season that brings beautiful colors back to nature. Spring is also the time to celebrate mothers, and Mother's Day is one of the sweetest days of the year. Karen and her mother, Doreen, appear together to show the true beauty of their bond.

DAUGHTER
KAREN

Karen, 54, was born in Washington, DC, but raised in Jamaica and Toronto. A graduate of Brown University and the University of London, she is a content producer and integrative wellness practitioner on a mission to promote "empowered aging."

Are there any beauty tips or tricks your family members passed on to you that you still use?

Moisturize your skin!

How has the meaning of beauty changed for you through the years?

My understanding of beauty as a reflection of what's in my heart and soul has only strengthened throughout my life.

What are your daily beauty routines?

I hydrate with lots of water, eat healthful foods, keep stress at bay with yoga and qigong, go makeup-free when not modeling, cleanse, and moisturize with products whose ingredients come from nature.

Do you have any beauty wisdom for the next generation?

Discover who you uniquely are and treat that person as a priceless treasure.

What makes you feel beautiful, and what does beauty mean to you?

A healthy body, a clear conscience, and a heart filled with love make me feel beautiful. Beauty in my everyday life means being of service, sharing kindness, connecting with others, creating, learning, breathing, and being grateful.

What is your motto for life?

Walk in the light, and you will reflect light. Sunshine eventually breaks through clouds.

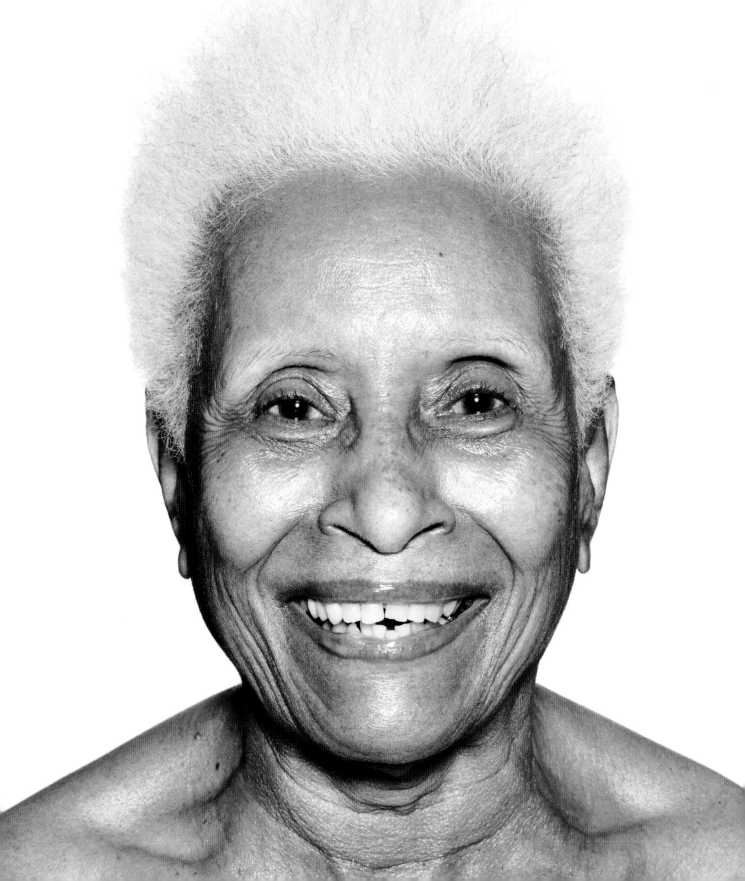

80 MOTHER DOREEN

Karen's mother, Doreen, 80, was born and raised in Jamaica. A graduate of Howard University, with a professional background in community development and counseling, she currently works part-time in Maryland. She is a firm believer in the value of work and service, especially when it helps empower others.

Are there any beauty tips or tricks your family members passed on to you that you still use?

My mother was an ardent believer in the benefits of moisturizing the skin.

How has the meaning of beauty changed for you through the years?

I was always told that beauty comes from within, and this belief has not changed.

What are your daily beauty routines?

I keep my skin clean and makeup-free (except for moisturizer and eyebrow pencil).

Do you have any beauty wisdom for the next generation?

Less is more. Keep it simple.

What makes you feel beautiful, and what does beauty mean to you?

Beauty is not something one earns; it's a gift. I choose to focus not on physical beauty but on what makes me feel alive, vital, and good. Music and dancing do that for me.

What is your motto for life?

Don't let anyone live "rent-free" in your head. Live fully in the present moment.

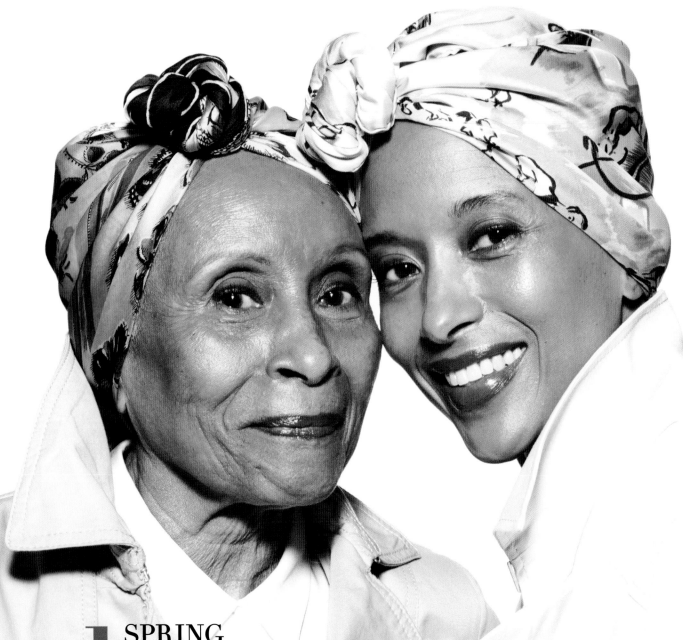

SPRING
day

I wanted to keep Karen's spring daytime look super simple. We first gave her a spray of rose water to refresh her foundation and add a hydrating layer.

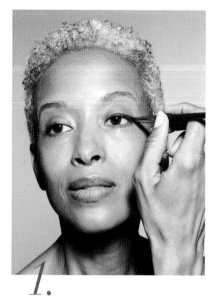

1.

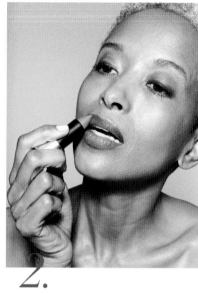

2.

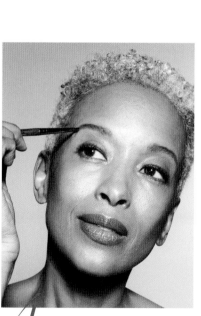

3.

4.

1. Karen used a small round brush (#7 on page 25) to line her eyes with dark lilac matte eye shadow.

2. She applied pink sheer lipstick for a hint of color and a really fresh look.

3. She then applied cream blush to the apples of her cheeks with a latex-free triangle-shaped sponge.

4. Karen used a brow brush (#10) to apply brow gel and fill in her eyebrows with a powdered shadow. She also applied mascara.

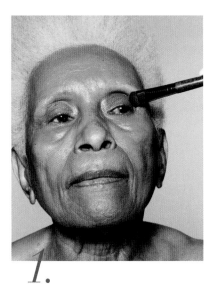 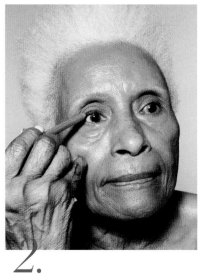 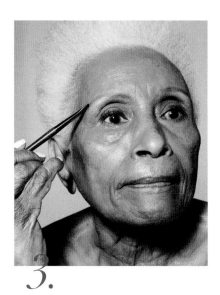

1.

2.

3.

SPRING
day

I wanted to create a beautiful spring palette on Doreen's face in colors that work well with her skin tone. It is important to leave the skin looking dewy, so it reflects light and looks the most natural and radiant. I used powder only on the eyelids and a bit on the forehead.

1. Rose-pink matte eye shadow was applied on the lids with a large round brush (#8 on page 25).

2. Lilac pencil liner works beautifully with the eye shadow color. Because Doreen's eyelids are big, I wanted the line to be thicker than usual. She blended the liner with a small round brush (#7).

3. After applying waterproof mascara, Doreen filled her brows with powdered brow color using an eyebrow brush (#10).

4. She used a latex-free triangle-shaped sponge to apply fresh pink cream blush on the apples of her cheeks, then blended well.

5. Doreen lined her lips before applying lipstick. Lip liner ensures that your lipstick stays put and makes the lips look even more defined.

6. Lipstick was applied straight from the tube. I chose a sheer texture for a light and fresh look.

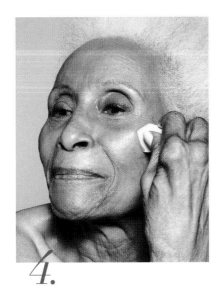

4.

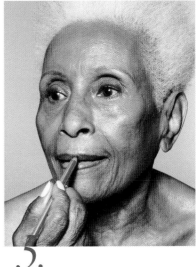

5.

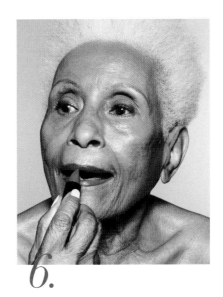

6.

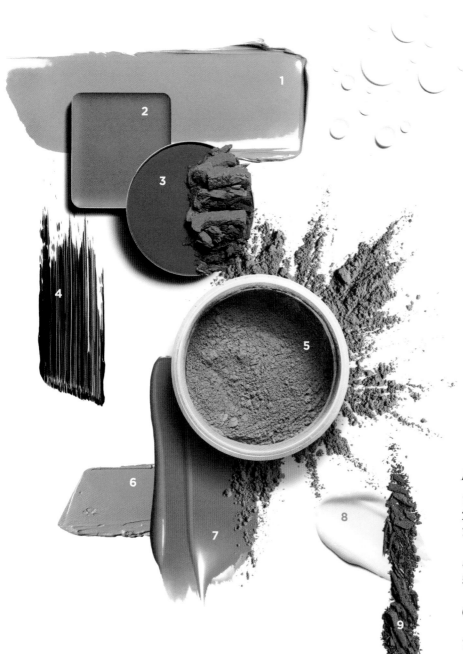

KAREN'S DAY products

1. Sheer lipstick
2. Cream blush
3. Matte eye shadow (used as eyeliner)
4. Waterproof mascara
5. Loose powder (dusted on the eyelids, forehead, and chin)
6. Concealer (smoothed over the eyelids and under the eyes)
7. Tinted moisturizer
8. Brow gel
9. Powdered brow color

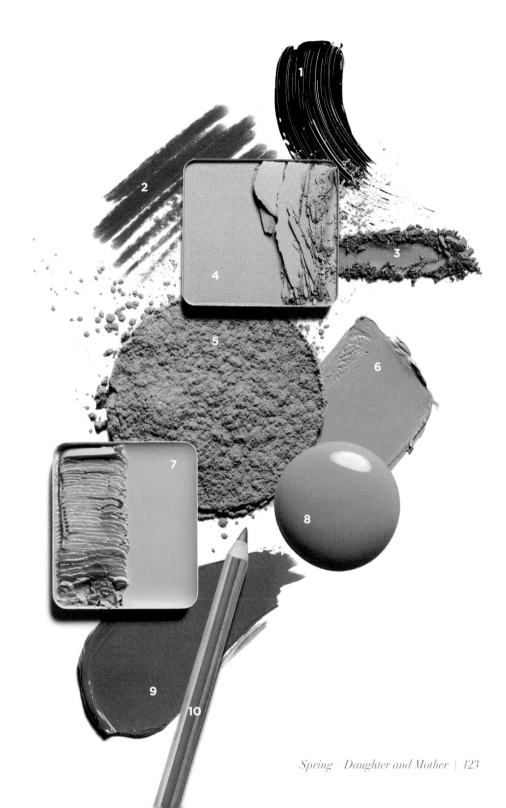

DOREEN'S DAY
products

1. Waterproof mascara
2. Eyeliner pencil
3. Powdered brow color
4. Matte eye shadow
5. Loose powder
6. Concealer (smoothed over the eyelids and under the eyes)
7. Cream blush
8. Light hydrating foundation
9. Sheer lipstick
10. Lip liner

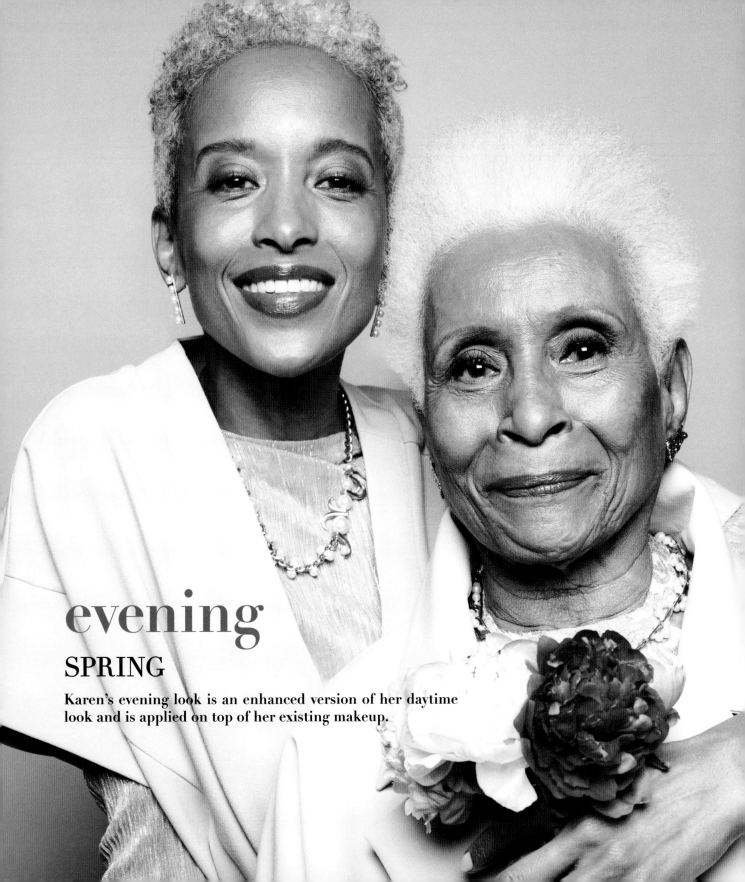

evening

SPRING

Karen's evening look is an enhanced version of her daytime look and is applied on top of her existing makeup.

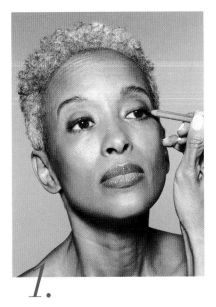

1.

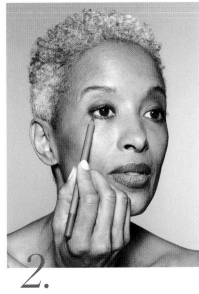

2.

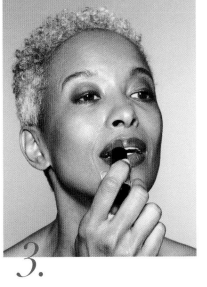

3.

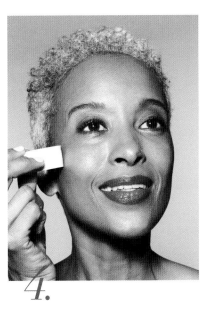

4.

1. Bright blue eyeliner pencil is applied on the upper lash line for a pop of color. Afterward, Karen blended this with a small brush (#7 on page 25).

2. She then applied pencil liner on her lower lash lines and on the waterlines.

3. Orange-red sheer lipstick goes well with blue eyeliner. She applied it straight from the tube so it would look natural and fresh.

4. She applied coral cream blush on the apples of her cheeks with a latex-free triangle-shaped sponge.

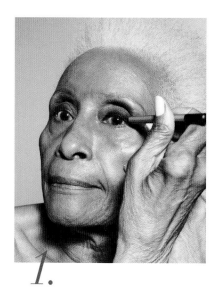 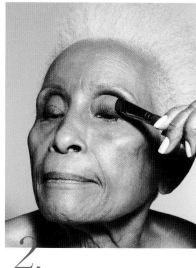 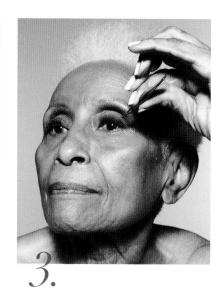

1.

2.

3.

evening

SPRING

I wanted to keep Doreen's evening color palette the same as her day palette but add more glamour, so we simply applied her evening look on top of her day look. I used a tiny bit of loose powder on Doreen's forehead and chin, but I wanted her skin to be dewy and fresh.

1. Doreen applied black eyeliner pencil on the top lash line.

2. She applied a pink matte eye shadow (brighter than the one she used for daytime) with a large round brush (#8 on page 25). Then she added purple matte eye shadow on the socket of the lids and on the outer corner of the eyes and blended.

3. She added individual short false eyelashes to make her lashes look thicker. This gives instant glam to the face.

4. Doreen then did a powder touch-up for the day-to-night transition.

5. She used a bright fuchsia lip liner to line and fill the lips.

6. Then she applied a pink cream blush on the apples of her cheeks with a latex-free triangle-shaped sponge.

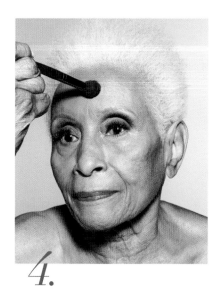

4.

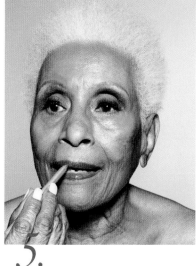

5.

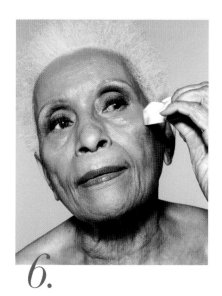

6.

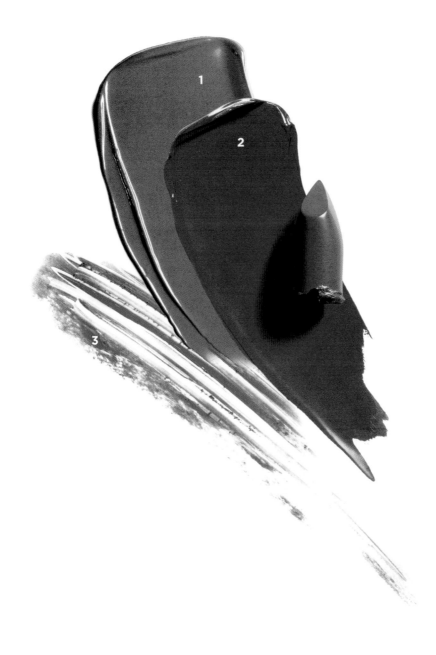

KAREN'S EVENING
products

1. Cream blush
2. Sheer lipstick
3. Eyeliner pencil

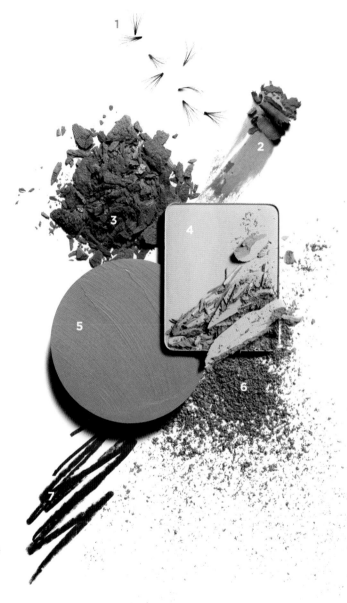

DOREEN'S EVENING
products

1. Individual short false eyelashes
2. Lip liner
3. Eye shadow #2
4. Eye shadow #1
5. Cream blush
6. Loose powder
7. Eyeliner pencil

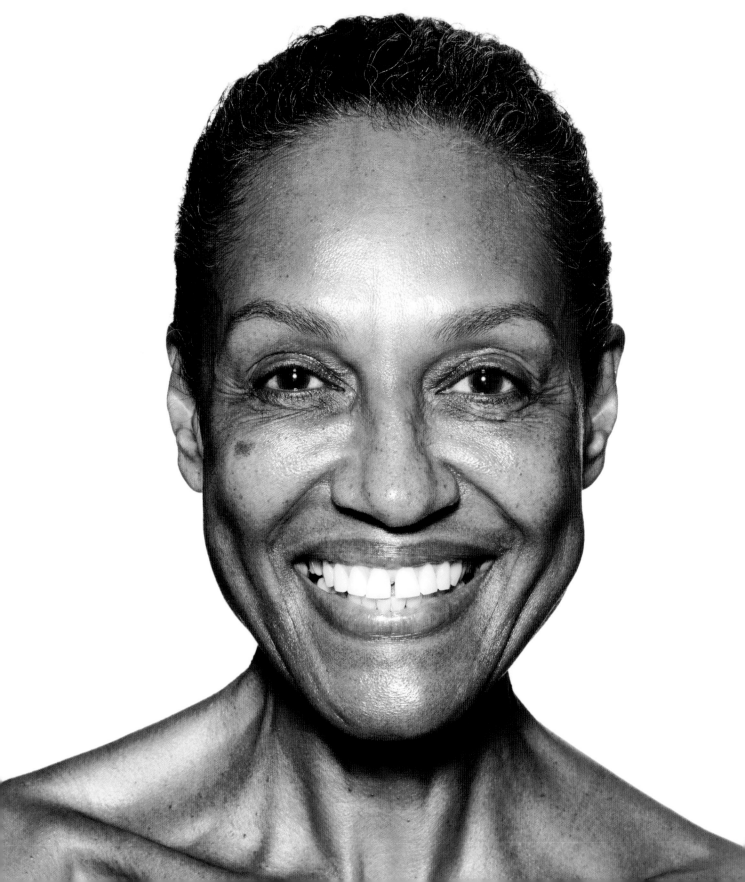

SUMMER IN SAINT-TROPEZ
PAT

The Caribbean beauty Pat, 65, is a photographer who likes theater, culture, meeting new people, and traveling the world.

Are there any beauty tips or tricks your family members passed on to you that you still use?

Living in the Caribbean during the First and Second World Wars, my grandmother and mother didn't have access to modern-day creams and potions. Coconut oil was by necessity their elixir of choice. It was their moisturizer, hair conditioner, body lotion, and, often, cooking oil. To this day I use it as a makeup remover and run the excess through my hair.

How has the meaning of beauty changed for you through the years?

When I was younger, my idea of beauty was having perfect skin and flashing, bright eyes. Today my idea of beauty is being comfortable in my own skin and having the light of happiness and kindness in my eyes.

What are your daily beauty routines?

I try to get a good night's sleep, drink lots of water, exercise, meditate, and center myself. I use eye cream and moisturizer with sunscreen on my face, and for my body I use any enriched body lotion that contains shea butter or cocoa butter. That's it.

Do you have any beauty wisdom for the next generation?

Diet, exercise, fresh air, and water are important. Always take your makeup off and nourish your skin with a good moisturizer before going to bed. Invest in good habits now!

What makes you feel beautiful, and what does beauty mean to you?

Beauty is coupled with strength and balance: to appreciate and be appreciated, to have gratitude, and to look out on life and say, "Take me or leave as I am—I have tried my best to rise to the occasion and make a positive impact."

What is your motto for life?

Onward and upward always. Believe!

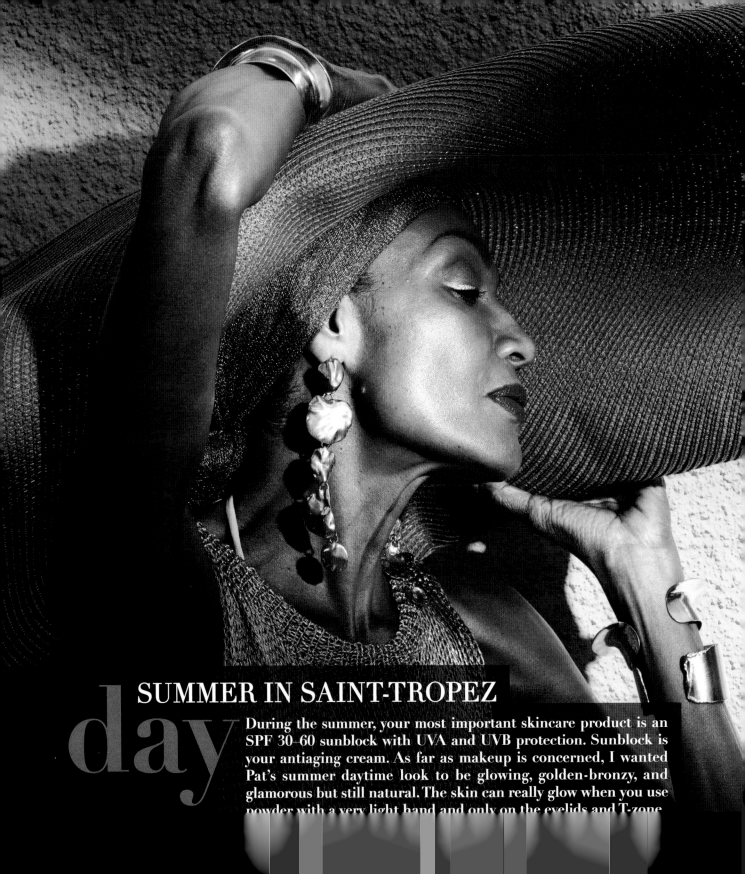

SUMMER IN SAINT-TROPEZ

day During the summer, your most important skincare product is an SPF 30–60 sunblock with UVA and UVB protection. Sunblock is your antiaging cream. As far as makeup is concerned, I wanted Pat's summer daytime look to be glowing, golden-bronzy, and glamorous but still natural. The skin can really glow when you use powder with a very light hand and only on the eyelids and T-zone

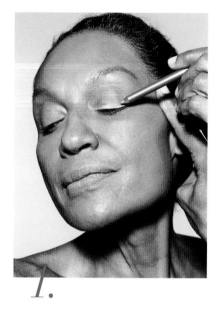

1.

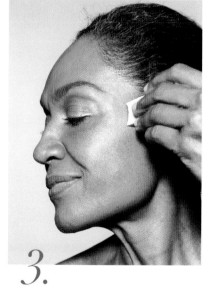

2.

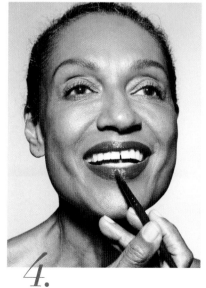

3.

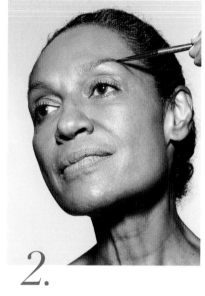

4.

1. Pat started her makeup by lining her upper lash line with a golden waterproof eye pencil, which lights up her entire face.

2. She filled and darkened her brows with brown shadow and a brow brush (#10 on page 25).

3. Pat used a latex-free triangle-shaped sponge to tap bronze liquid highlighter on her cheeks, accentuating her bone structure and adding a touch of glamour.

4. I chose a beautiful deep terra-cotta hydrating cream lipstick, which complements Pat's outfit and makeup perfectly. Applying it with a lip brush allows her to create a sharp outline.

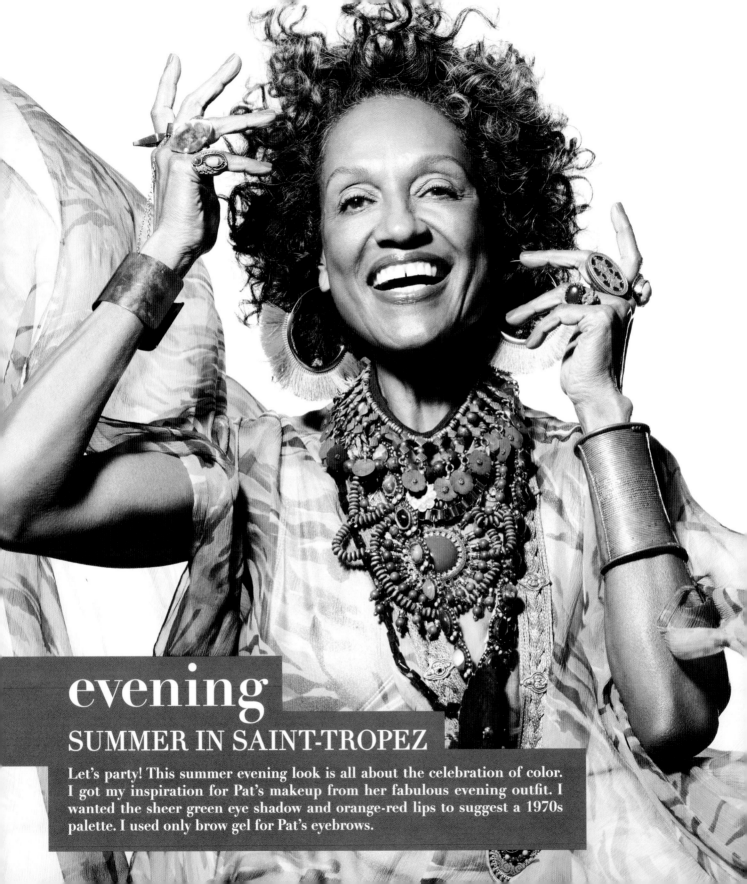

evening
SUMMER IN SAINT-TROPEZ

Let's party! This summer evening look is all about the celebration of color. I got my inspiration for Pat's makeup from her fabulous evening outfit. I wanted the sheer green eye shadow and orange-red lips to suggest a 1970s palette. I used only brow gel for Pat's eyebrows.

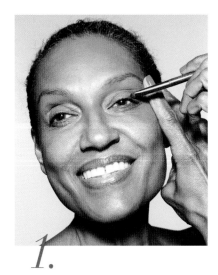

1.

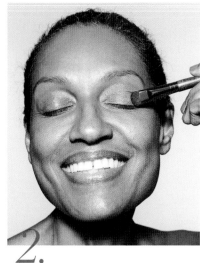

2.

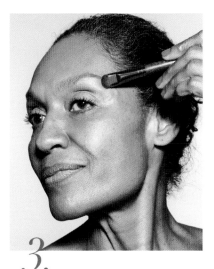

1. Pat started her makeup by applying bright green semimatte eye shadow to the roots of her lashes with a small round brush (#7 on page 25).

2. Then she applied the same green shadow all over the lids up to the crease with a large round brush (#8) and blended well.

3. A lighter green shadow was applied under the brow bone to create more light and that true '70s disco feel.

4. Pat applied bright orange cream blush to her cheeks with a latex-free triangle-shaped sponge.

5. Coral sheer lipstick looks fresh and goes well with the rest of Pat's makeup. She applied it straight from the tube.

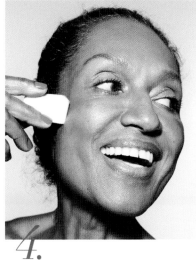

3.

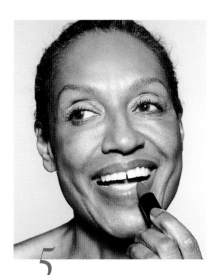

4.

Summer in Saint-Tropez | 135

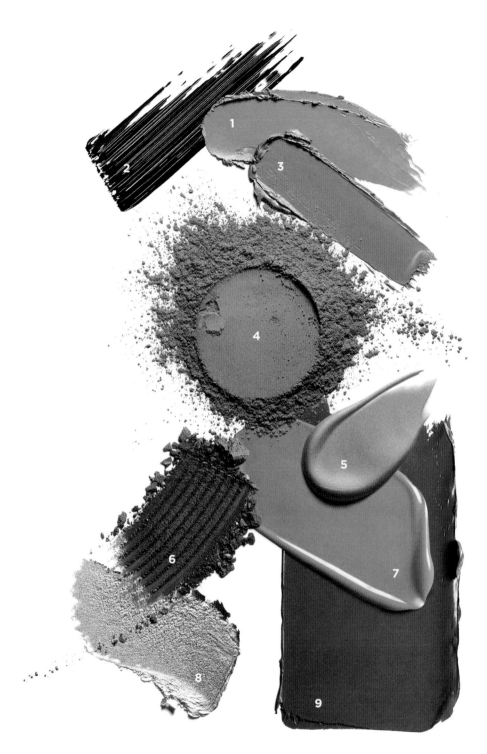

DAY products

1. Color corrector
2. Waterproof mascara
3. Concealer
4. Loose powder
5. Bronze highlighter
6. Brow color
7. Tinted moisturizer
8. Eyeliner pencil
9. Cream lipstick

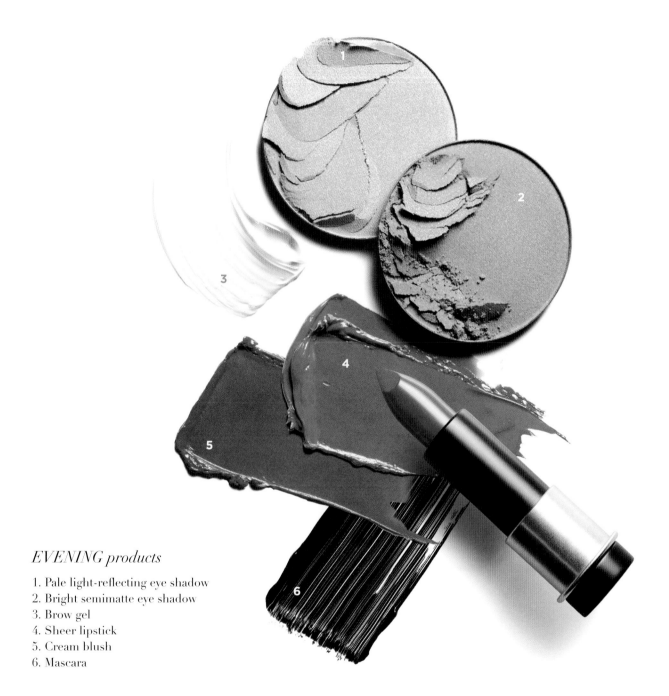

EVENING *products*

1. Pale light-reflecting eye shadow
2. Bright semimatte eye shadow
3. Brow gel
4. Sheer lipstick
5. Cream blush
6. Mascara

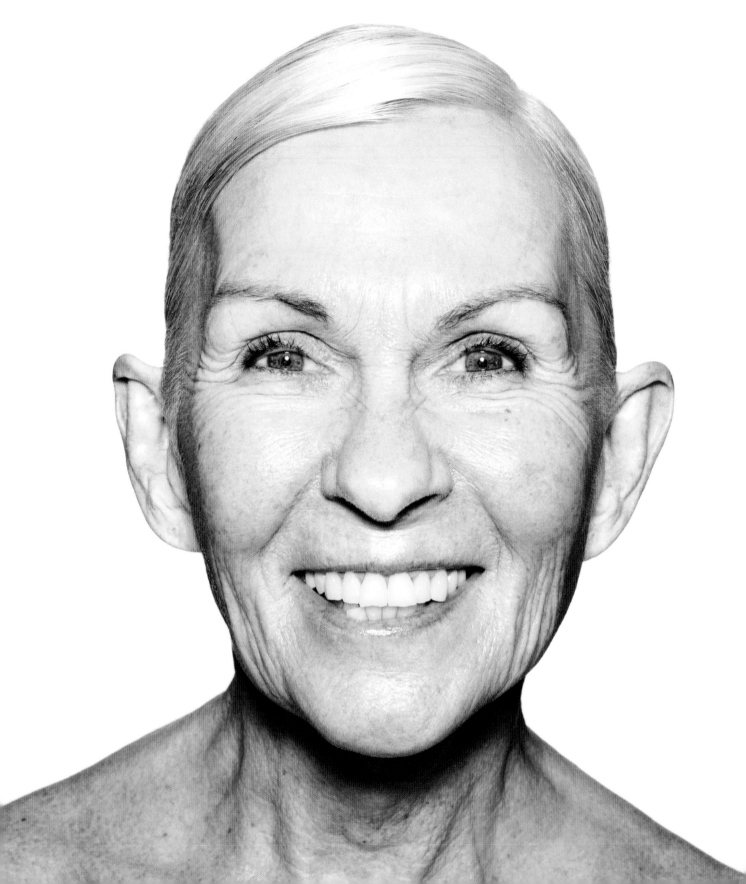

64
AUTUMN IN NEW YORK
MAARIT

Finnish-born Manhattan resident Maarit, 64, travels with her husband around the world and spends the summer months with her family at their homes in southern France and Finland. Maarit loves to dress up and express herself through beautiful clothes and accessories.

Are there any beauty tips or tricks your family members passed on to you that you still use?

Never go to bed without cleaning your face and teeth.

How has the meaning of beauty changed for you through the years?

When I was younger, people focused on the surface when talking about beauty, but now they consider the whole package—style, confidence, and humor.

What are your daily beauty routines?

To begin the day and to wake me up, I like rinsing my face with icy cold water before applying serum and day cream. I get daily exercise. I take a long walk in the morning in Central Park with my dog, then go to the gym, play tennis, or do Pilates.

Do you have any beauty wisdom for the next generation?

It scares me that people go for Botox and other fillers at increasingly younger ages, trying to create perfection. Often the results are the opposite.

What makes you feel beautiful?

I feel beautiful after a good, long night's sleep.

What is your motto for life?

I have two: what goes around comes around, and everyone creates their own happiness.

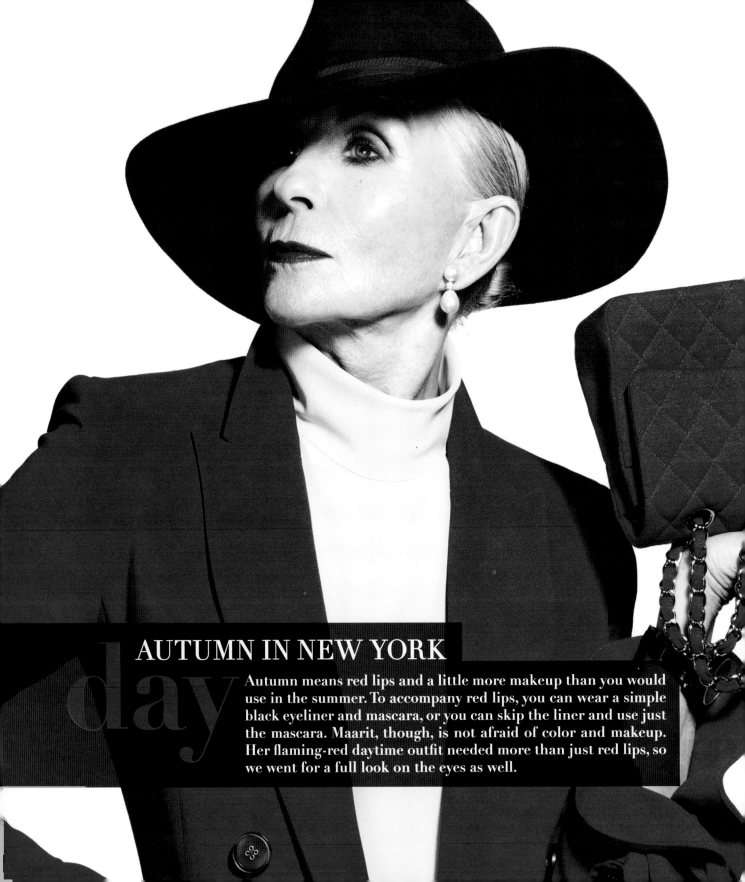

AUTUMN IN NEW YORK

day

Autumn means red lips and a little more makeup than you would use in the summer. To accompany red lips, you can wear a simple black eyeliner and mascara, or you can skip the liner and use just the mascara. Maarit, though, is not afraid of color and makeup. Her flaming-red daytime outfit needed more than just red lips, so we went for a full look on the eyes as well.

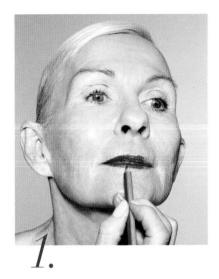

1.

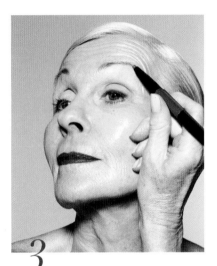

3.

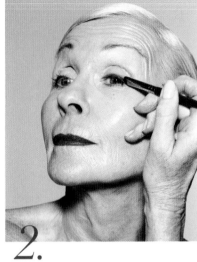

2.

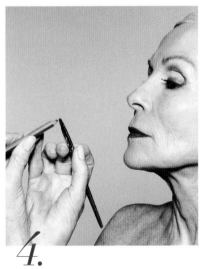

4.

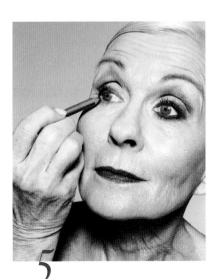

5.

1. Sometimes it's a good idea to make up your lips first instead of your eyes. That way you can see how much more makeup you need. Maarit used red lip pencil, so the result is very matte — it stays well during lunch meetings. You just need to moisturize your lips beforehand.

2. I chose a dark turquoise pencil to line Maarit's upper lash line. She blended it with a small round brush (#7 on page 25).

3. Maarit then lightly filled in her eyebrows with a brown brow pencil.

4. I taught Maarit how to rub the pencil color onto her eye shadow brush so it's easier to apply the color on the crease of the eyelid as well as on the lower lash line. Afterward, she used the brush to blend well. The dark turquoise color lightens up to an icy blue.

5. She also used the eyeliner pencil on the lower and upper waterlines. She used a dark midnight-blue matte eye shadow to darken the lash lines, too, giving depth to the eyes.

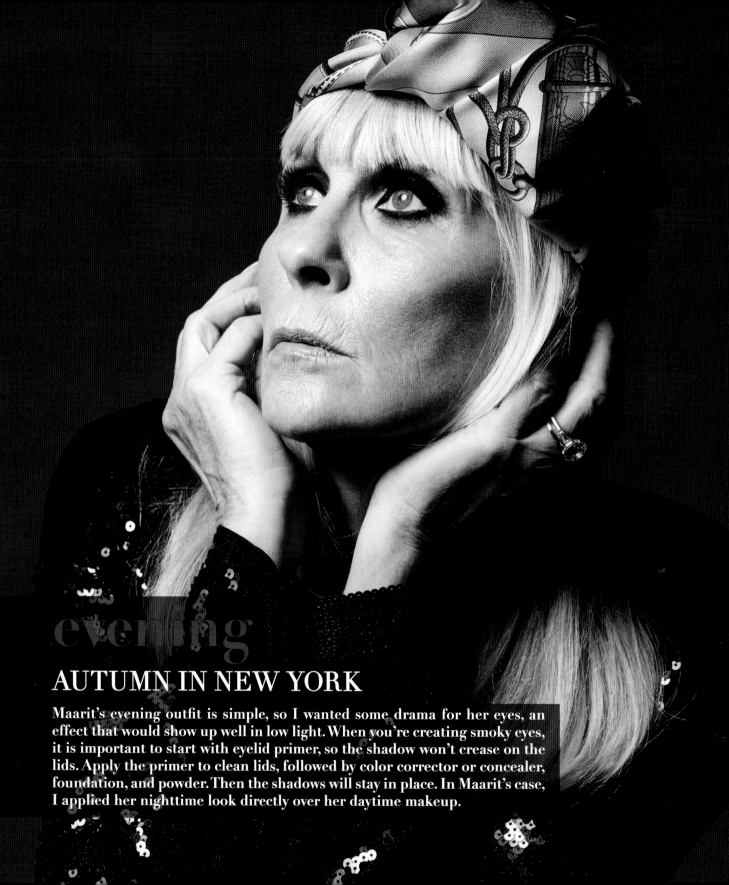

AUTUMN IN NEW YORK

Maarit's evening outfit is simple, so I wanted some drama for her eyes, an effect that would show up well in low light. When you're creating smoky eyes, it is important to start with eyelid primer, so the shadow won't crease on the lids. Apply the primer to clean lids, followed by color corrector or concealer, foundation, and powder. Then the shadows will stay in place. In Maarit's case, I applied her nighttime look directly over her daytime makeup.

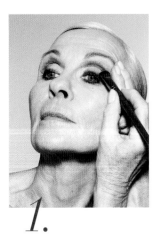

1.

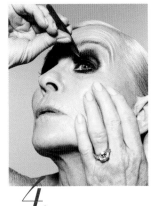

2.

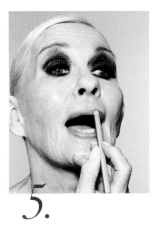

3.

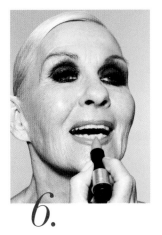

4.

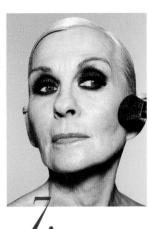

5.

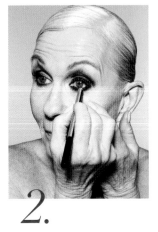

6.

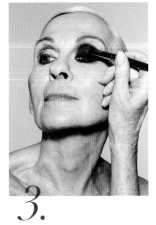

7.

1. Maarit applied black matte eye shadow to the roots of her upper lashes with a small round brush (#7 on page 25) and blended well with a large round brush (#8).

2. Here she lined the upper and lower lash lines with black eyeliner. She blended well, then filled in the waterline with black liner.

3. Using a large round brush (#8), she applied black eye shadow all over the lids and in the crease. She tapped the brush a couple of times on the container to remove excess shadow so it wouldn't land on her cheeks.

4. Maarit likes full false eyelashes for her evening looks. She let the adhesive dry on the strips for twenty seconds, then applied them to the lash line with tweezers.

5. I chose a light peach lip liner, which Maarit applied before the lipstick. The wax of the liner creates a "wall" around the lips so the lipstick won't run into the small lines around the mouth.

6. Then she applied lipstick straight from the tube.

7. Even though I am not a big fan of contouring, bronzer was the right choice for this look. She applied it with a blush brush (#6) to create warmth and bring out her high cheekbones.

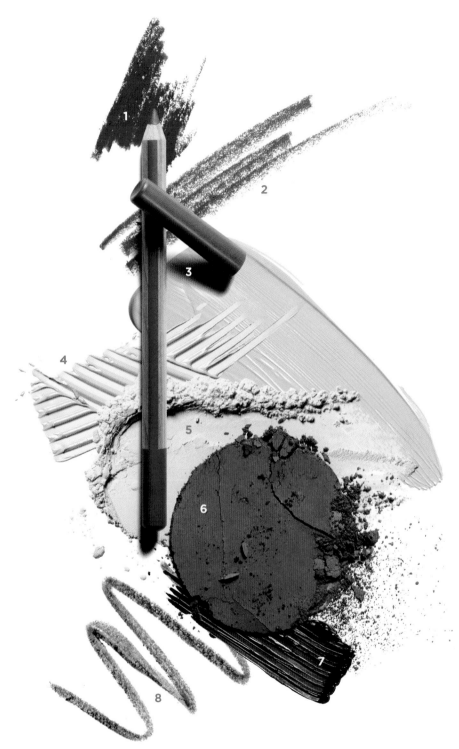

DAY products

1. Lip liner
2. Brow pencil
3. Light hydrating foundation
4. Concealer
5. Transparent loose powder
   (applied to the eyelids and
   middle of the forehead)
6. Matte eye shadow
7. Waterproof mascara
8. Eyeliner pencil

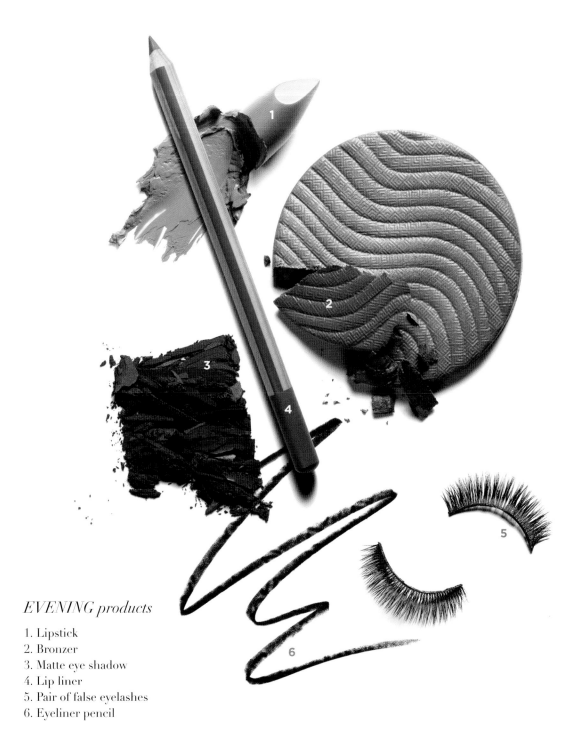

EVENING products

1. Lipstick
2. Bronzer
3. Matte eye shadow
4. Lip liner
5. Pair of false eyelashes
6. Eyeliner pencil

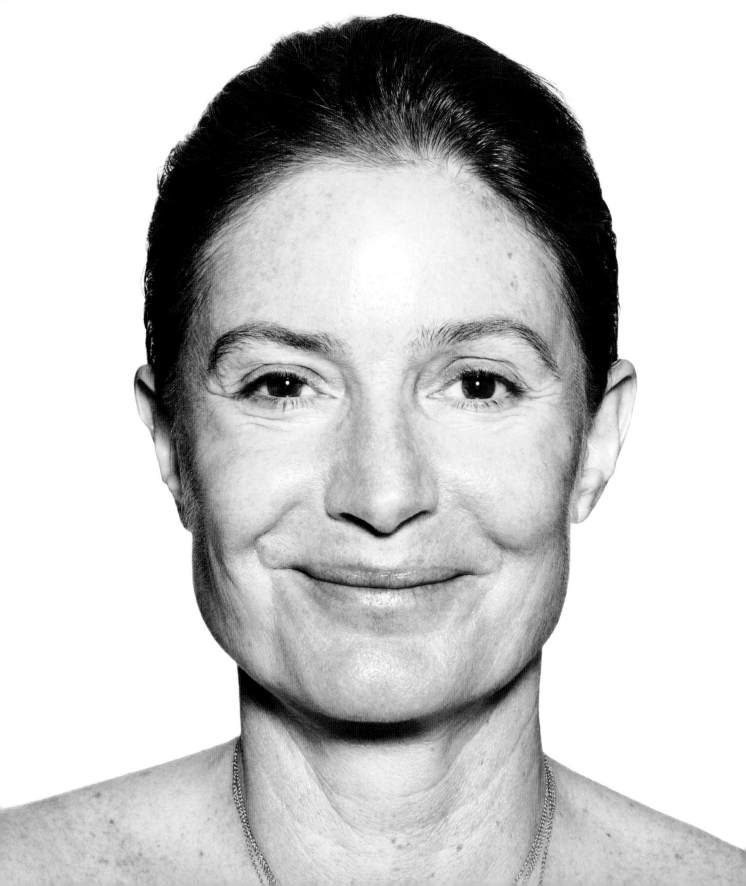

WINTER FASHION
CELINE

French-born fashion and beauty PR master Celine, 50, is a tastemaker and a connoisseur of all things French and chic. Celine loves fashion and dressing up as much she loves traveling. Her trademarks are her flaming-red hair and her many big rings, which she never takes off.

Are there any beauty tips or tricks your family members passed on to you that you still use?

My beloved grandmother taught me to fortify, enrich, and whiten my nails by dipping them in lemon halves and to pinch my cheeks for an instant glow.

How has the meaning of beauty changed for you through the years?

Beauty means beauty inside and out. It means healthy skin. Beauty also means business to me, as I do PR for French cosmetics brands.

What are your daily beauty routines?

It's all about the skin, really. Cleanliness and hydration are the most important elements for me. I apply light face serums at night and go for deep-cleansing facials regularly.

Do you have any beauty wisdom for the next generation?

Be yourself. Find your strengths and learn how to take care of them—hair, skin, smile, teeth, eyes . . . whatever they might be.

What makes you feel beautiful?

It's terrible to say, but I love when my skin feels sunkissed. I also am happiest when I feel skinny, so exercising makes me happy!

What is your motto for life?

One day at a time. Listen and learn.

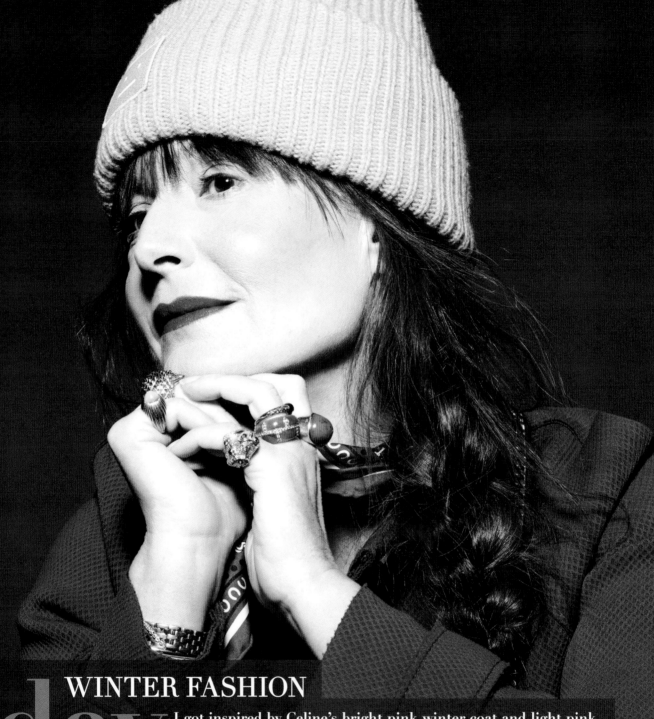

WINTER FASHION

day

I got inspired by Celine's bright pink winter coat and light pink beanie. I wanted her makeup to look modern and cool without making it seem like she was trying too hard.

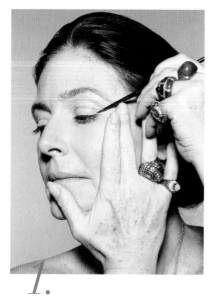

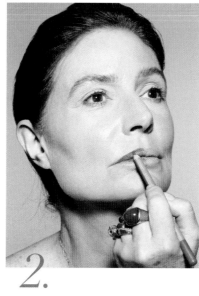

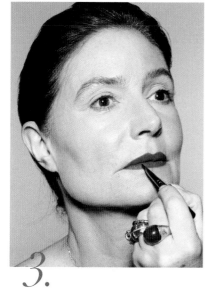

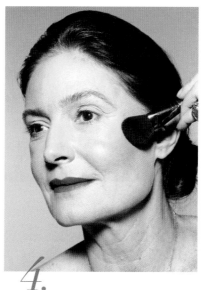

1. I chose a bright yellow waterproof eyeliner that gives a bit of an edge. Using an eyeliner brush (#11 on page 25), Celine drew a line across the top of her lashes and extended it to the inner corners of her eyes. She didn't apply any mascara—she just let the eyeliner work its magic.

2. After Celine's lips were moisturized, she tapped foundation on them to provide a good base for her lip color. She then lined and filled her lips with an orange-red lip pencil.

3. Celine applied bright orange-red matte lipstick with a lip brush (#12), which gave her very sharp lip lines. The color combination of yellow eyeliner and orange-red lips is quite electric.

4. Using a powder brush (#6), she applied peach blush to her cheeks, just below the apples, to create a natural contour. Blush is very important in winter to give a hint of color to the face.

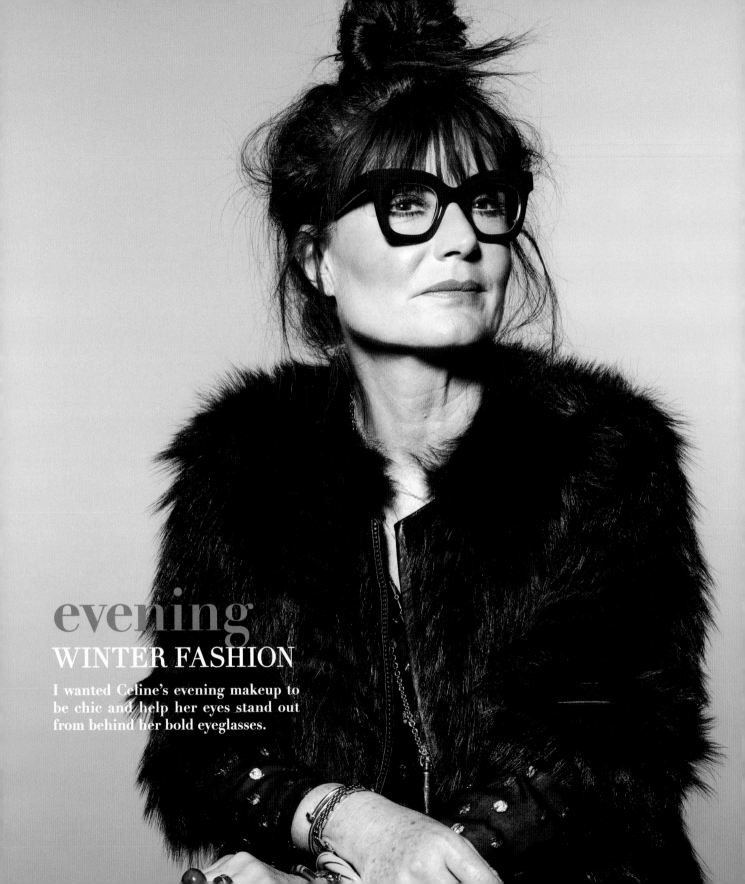

evening
WINTER FASHION

I wanted Celine's evening makeup to be chic and help her eyes stand out from behind her bold eyeglasses.

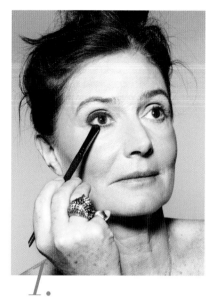

1.

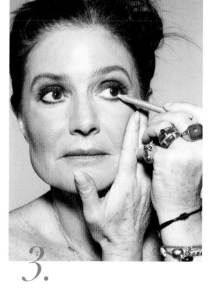

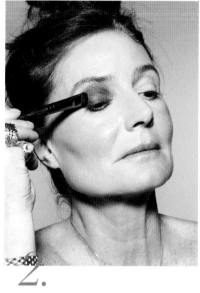

2.

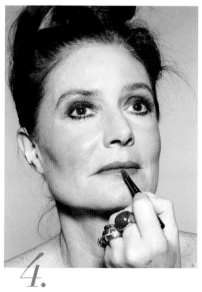

3.

4.

1. Celine applied a brown-bronze matte eye shadow on the upper and lower lash lines using a small round brush (#7 on page 25).

2. Then, using a blending brush (#8), she blended the shadow all over her lids, up to the crease.

3. Using white eye pencil on the waterline is an old Hollywood makeup trick that makes your eyes look bigger. It also helps when you're wearing eyeglasses.

4. Soft lips with strong eyes look modern and cool. I chose a light coral-pink cream lipstick that was applied with the help of a lip brush (#12).

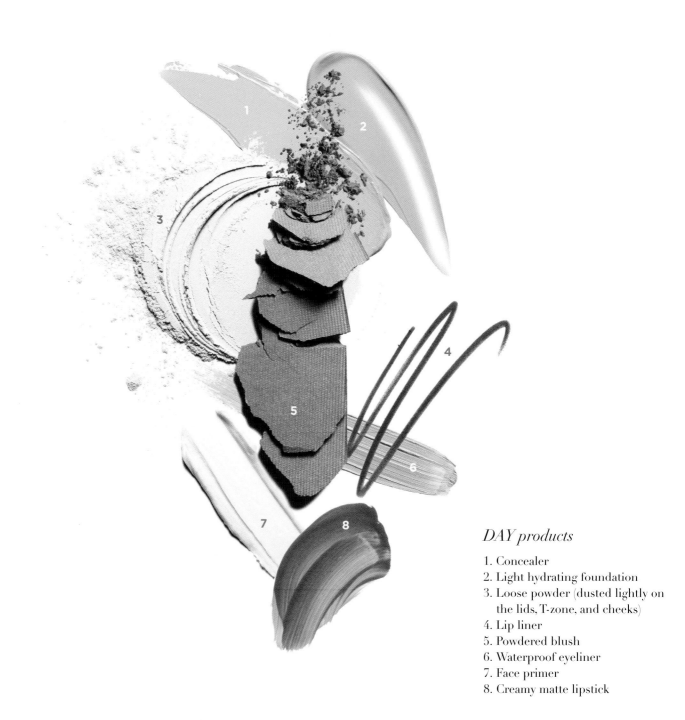

DAY products

1. Concealer
2. Light hydrating foundation
3. Loose powder (dusted lightly on the lids, T-zone, and cheeks)
4. Lip liner
5. Powdered blush
6. Waterproof eyeliner
7. Face primer
8. Creamy matte lipstick

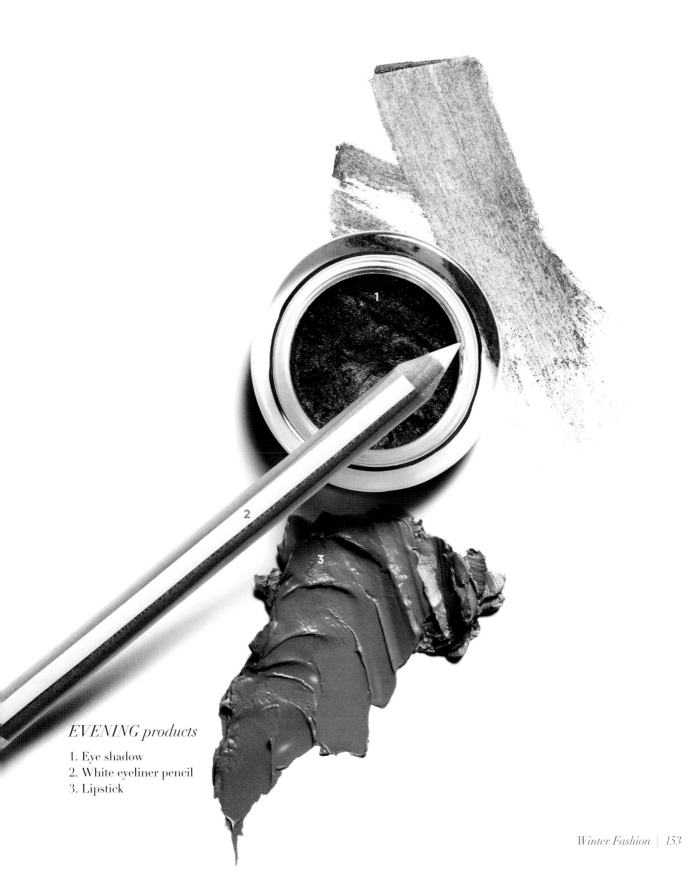

EVENING products

1. Eye shadow
2. White eyeliner pencil
3. Lipstick

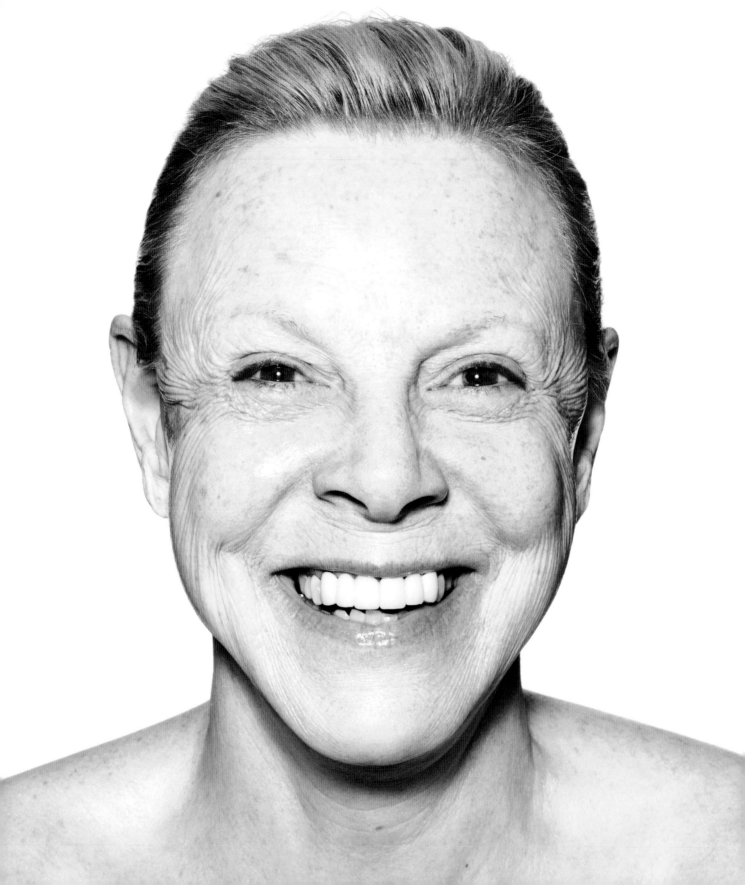

HOLLYWOOD GLAMOUR SIOBHAN

Siobhan, 66, has always been interested in neuroscience and psychology and works as a reflexologist. In her free time, she bakes, watches old black-and-white movies, attends the theater, and goes dancing. She loves to laugh and have a good time.

Are there any beauty tips or tricks your family members passed on to you that you still use?

My mother taught me the importance of blending foundation over your face, neck, and ears as well as the importance of choosing the right color for your skin tone.

How has the meaning of beauty changed for you through the years?

When I was young, beauty was about drama. I wanted to accentuate my features, my makeup. Today, for me, beauty is elegance.

What are your daily beauty routines?

In the morning I tap my face with cold water. Then I apply moisturizer and a combination foundation and sunscreen. At night I use an organic, fragrance-free wipe to take off my makeup. I also dampen a wash-cloth, pour raw unfiltered honey onto it, and use it to gently wash my face, neck, and ears. Then I put moisturizer on my face and body.

Do you have any beauty wisdom for the next generation?

Smile!

What does beauty mean to you?

Being happy with who I am. Being true to who I am. Everyday beauty is putting on makeup, fixing my hair, and dressing as me—Siobhan. And being positive toward myself and others.

What is your motto for life?

Live from the heart—with vulnerability, compassion, kindness, empathy, lots of laughter, and fun.

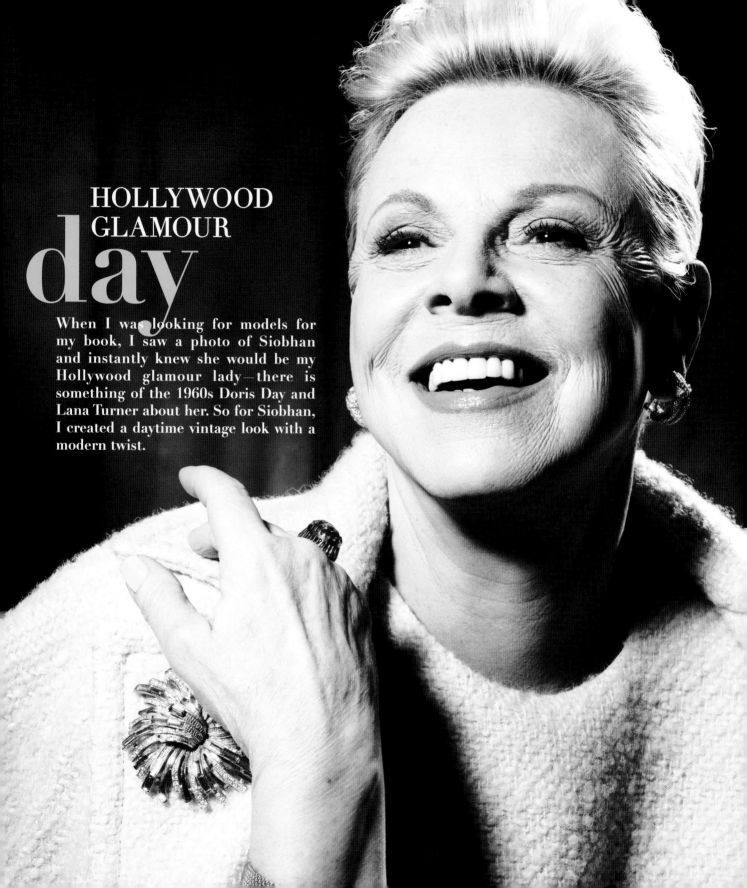

HOLLYWOOD GLAMOUR
day

When I was looking for models for my book, I saw a photo of Siobhan and instantly knew she would be my Hollywood glamour lady—there is something of the 1960s Doris Day and Lana Turner about her. So for Siobhan, I created a daytime vintage look with a modern twist.

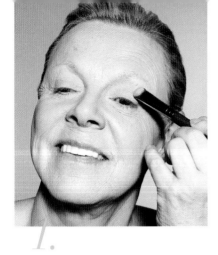

1.

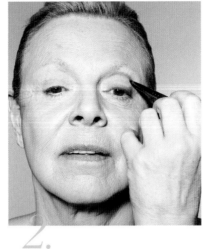

2.

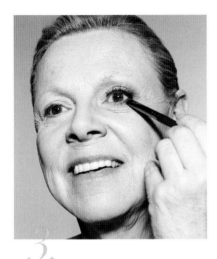

3.

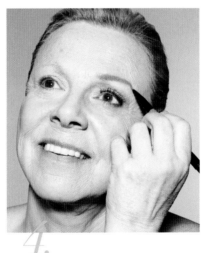

4.

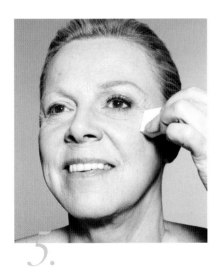

5.

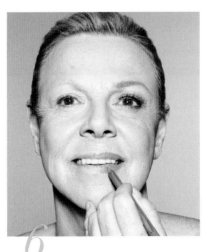

6.

1. Siobhan started her eye makeup by using a large round brush (#8 on page 25) to apply a light beige-pink matte eye shadow on the eyelids up to the crease. This color works as a base that creates light on the eyes and makes a good canvas for the rest of the shadows.

2. Using a small round brush (#7), she applied light brown matte eye shadow—not shimmery, because that would look dated during the daytime—on the roots of the upper lash line and on the crease. Then she used a large round brush (#8) to blend.

3. Dark brown eyeliner pencil is a softer choice for daytime than classic black. Siobhan started from the outer corner and drew a line to the inner corner, but only over the line where her lashes grow. She also applied it to the outer corner of the bottom lash line, used a brush to blend, then applied mascara.

4. Siobhan filled in her eyebrows with pencil in a light taupe color.

5. Cream blush keeps makeup looking fresh and skin dewy. Here she applied a rose-pink cream blush with a latex-free triangle-shaped sponge.

6. Siobhan covered her lips in foundation, then colored her lips with a warm, light-coral lip liner.

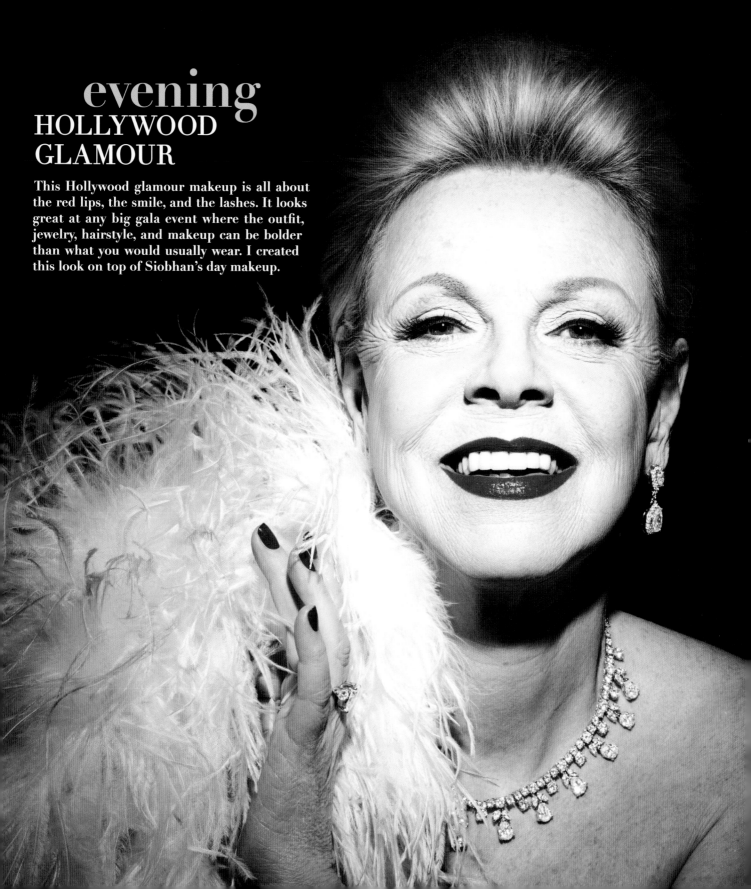

evening
HOLLYWOOD GLAMOUR

This Hollywood glamour makeup is all about the red lips, the smile, and the lashes. It looks great at any big gala event where the outfit, jewelry, hairstyle, and makeup can be bolder than what you would usually wear. I created this look on top of Siobhan's day makeup.

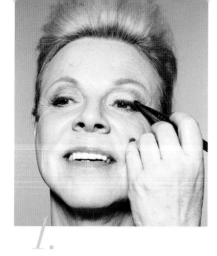

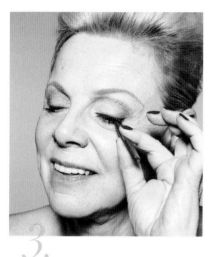

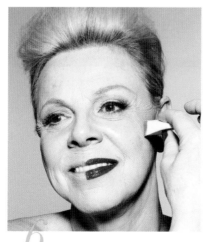

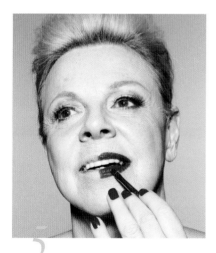

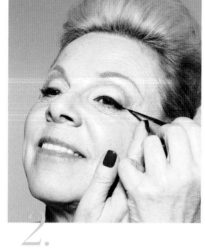

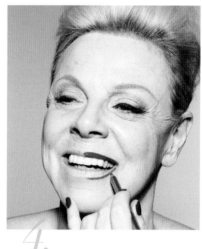

1. Siobhan applied white matte eye shadow on her lids with a small round brush (#7 on page 25) to open up her eyes and achieve an instant retro feel.

2. Classic black eyeliner gives the 1950s style more attitude. I like gel liners because they are less messy if you make a mistake. Using an eyeliner brush (#11), Siobhan extended the line into the familiar retro "wings."

3. Next, she attached false eyelashes at the outer corners of her eyes, which added volume and made her eyes look bigger. She used tweezers and let the adhesive dry around twenty seconds on the strips before she applied them.

4. Just as she did for her daytime look, Siobhan sponged foundation onto her lips to hide her natural undertone. Lip liner also builds a "wall" around the lips so the lipstick won't run into the fine lines around the mouth.

5. Red lipstick is a must. After lining and filling the lips, she applied matching red lipstick with a lip brush (#12). Siobhan was careful to stay within the boundaries established by the lip liner.

6. She applied pink cream blush to the apples of the cheeks using a latex-free triangle-shaped sponge.

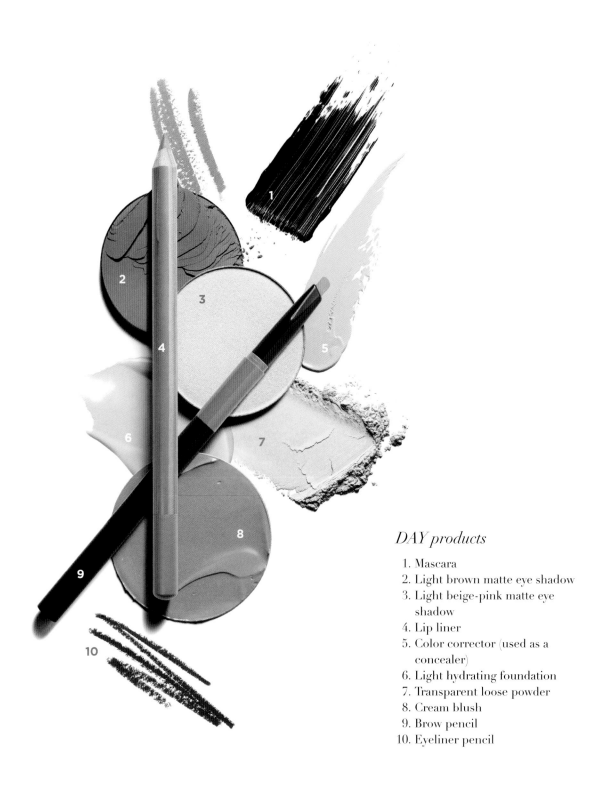

DAY products

1. Mascara
2. Light brown matte eye shadow
3. Light beige-pink matte eye shadow
4. Lip liner
5. Color corrector (used as a concealer)
6. Light hydrating foundation
7. Transparent loose powder
8. Cream blush
9. Brow pencil
10. Eyeliner pencil

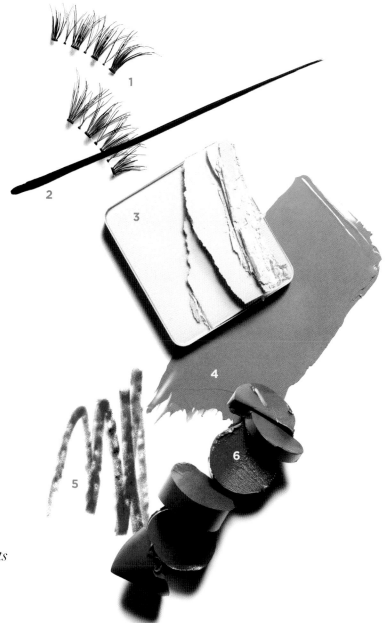

EVENING products

1. False eyelashes
2. Gel eyeliner
3. Matte eye shadow
4. Cream blush
5. Lip liner
6. Lipstick

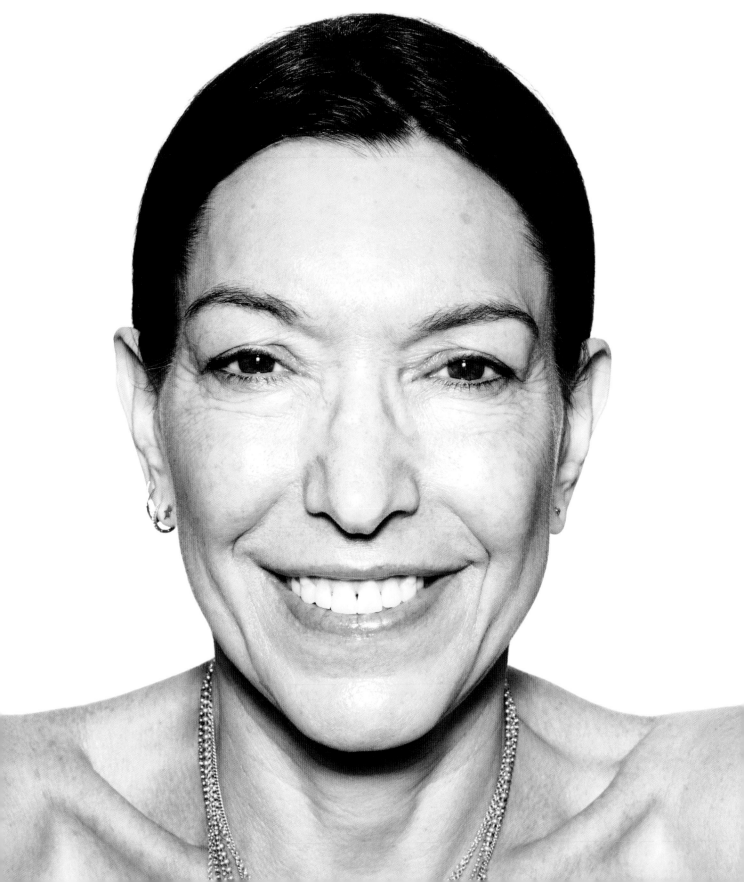

ROCKER CHIC
MIMI

Fashion stylist and costume designer Mimi, 57, is a die-hard native New Yorker whose style is inspired by the city's energy and vibrant cultural scene. She travels around the world for her assignments in the fashion and music industries. When she's not working, she spends as much time as possible with her family.

Are there any beauty tips or tricks your family members passed on to you that you still use?

Yes! My mother taught me how to take care of myself physically, mentally, and spiritually. She taught me to eat healthful, unprocessed plant-based foods; she taught me to exercise and meditate. Taking care of yourself is not superficial—it is empowering. My mother wears no makeup but uses face cream and sunblock year-round. She has inspired me to do the same. My grandmother washed her face with Dove soap and moisturized with Nivea cream at night. She never went out in the sun and had no wrinkles on her face. She also was adventurous with her makeup, and that had a huge influence on me.

How has the meaning of beauty changed for you through the years?

I don't think of beauty as being simply physical or about perfection. I think beauty is all about your attitude and feeling comfortable in your own skin. It's about being true to yourself and being happy, and it's about being a kind, loving, and giving person.

What are your daily beauty routines?

I meditate every day, then I exercise. And then . . . I put on tons of eyeliner. More is never enough!

Do you have any beauty wisdom for the next generation?

Be yourself; develop your own style; don't try too hard to be perfect. Have a sense of humor about your looks. Being kind makes you more beautiful than any makeup or product can.

What makes you feel beautiful?

Eyeliner, great shoes, and jewelry make me feel and look beautiful. Happiness is being around my family—my mother, my husband, and my two sons—and that makes me feel beautiful. Being helpful also makes me feel beautiful.

What is your motto for life?

Keep saying yes to things. Stay open to everything. Keep putting yourself out there and taking chances. Be fearless and badass.

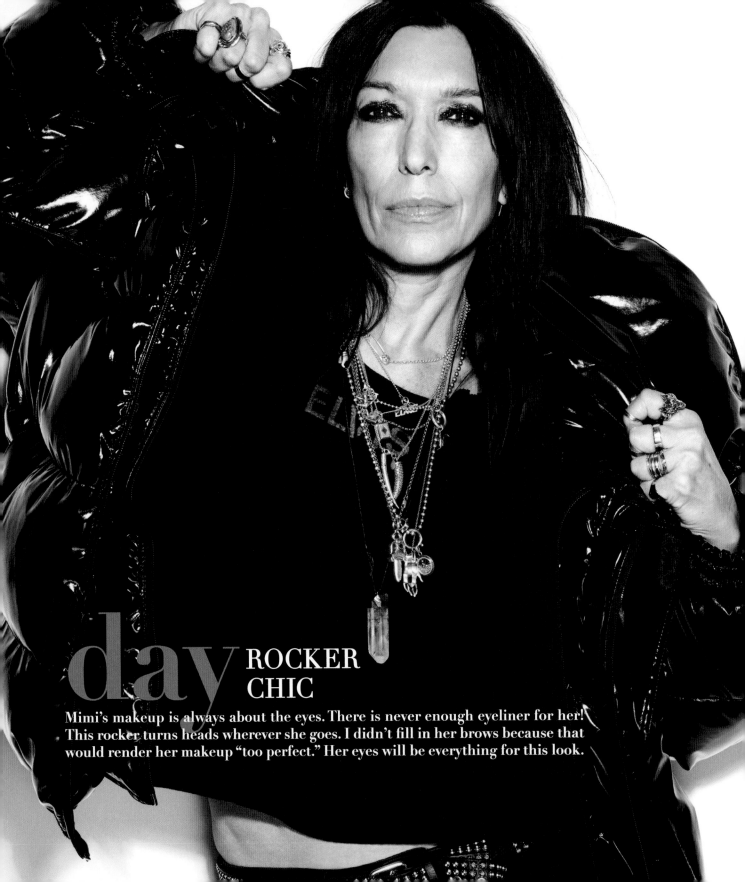

day ROCKER CHIC

Mimi's makeup is always about the eyes. There is never enough eyeliner for her! This rocker turns heads wherever she goes. I didn't fill in her brows because that would render her makeup "too perfect." Her eyes will be everything for this look.

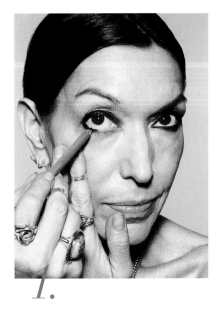

1.

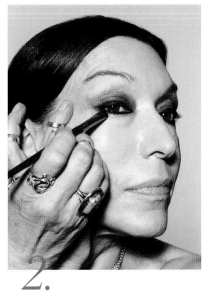

2.

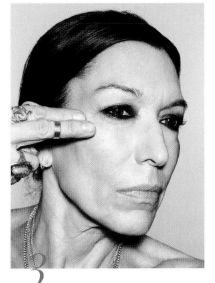

3.

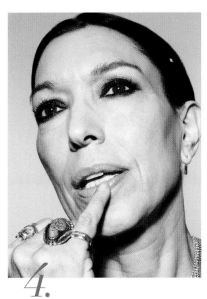

4.

1. Under the foundation, Mimi applied eyelid primer so her eye makeup would last longer. She applied black pencil liner to the upper and lower lash lines as well as on the waterline. She also added lots of mascara to her lashes. This creates a more intense effect.

2. She used an eye shadow brush (#7 on page 25) to blend the liners and make the eyes more smoky.

3. Then she applied Elizabeth Arden's Eight Hour Cream Skin Protectant on her cheeks and eyelids for a dewy look.

4. Finally, she applied Elizabeth Arden's Eight Hour Cream Skin Protectant on her lips.

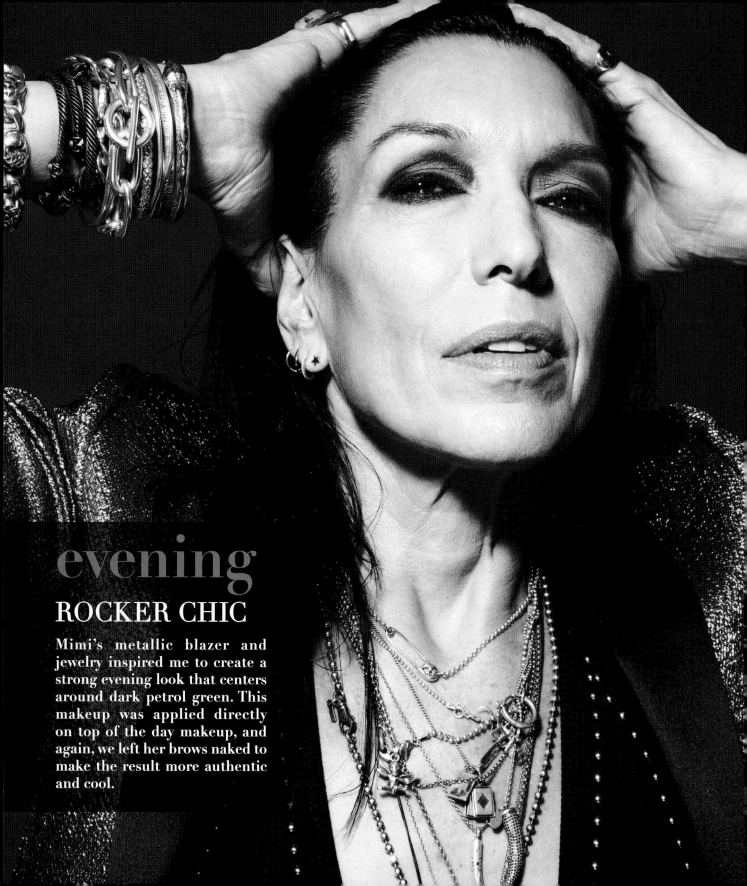

evening
ROCKER CHIC

Mimi's metallic blazer and jewelry inspired me to create a strong evening look that centers around dark petrol green. This makeup was applied directly on top of the day makeup, and again, we left her brows naked to make the result more authentic and cool.

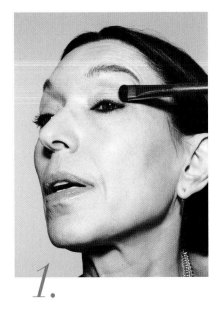

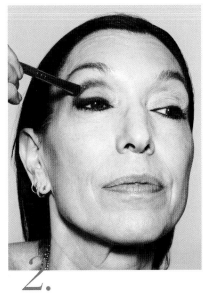

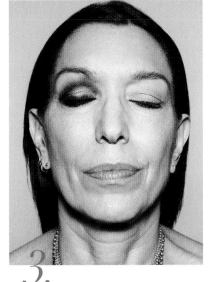

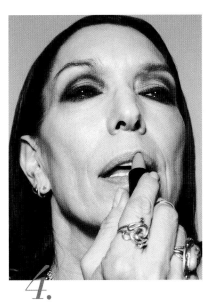

1. Mimi tapped transparent loose powder on her lids to give them a matte finish.

2. Using a small round brush (#7 on page 25), she applied dark petrol green matte eye shadow to the lash line and on the crease to accentuate her eyes.

3. After blending the color on the upper lid, Mimi added a lighter and more shimmery green on top of the dark shadow on the lower lash line. The shimmer on the lash line reflects the light.

4. A very light coral sheer lipstick was enough color for her lips.

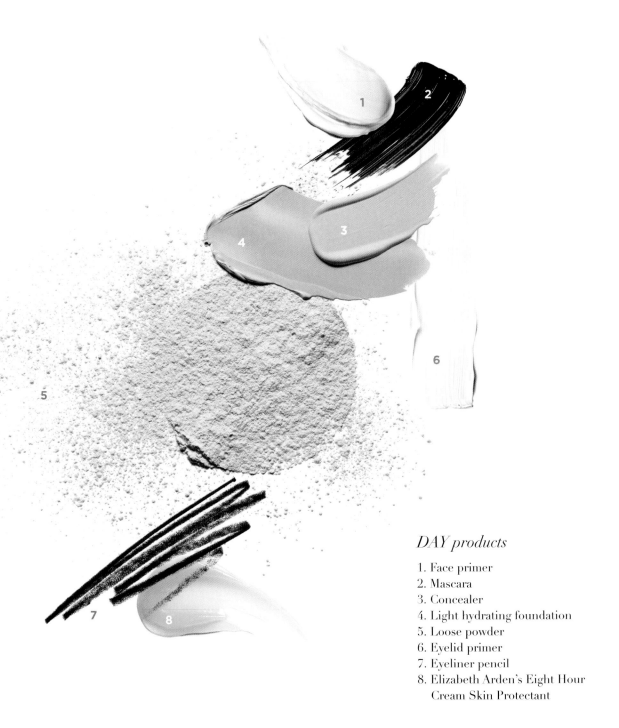

DAY products

1. Face primer
2. Mascara
3. Concealer
4. Light hydrating foundation
5. Loose powder
6. Eyelid primer
7. Eyeliner pencil
8. Elizabeth Arden's Eight Hour
   Cream Skin Protectant

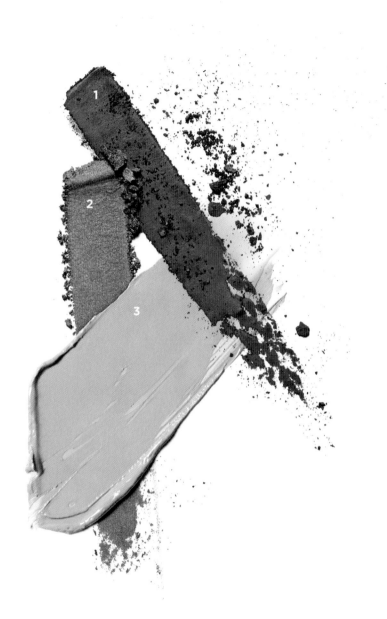

EVENING products

1. Dark matte eye shadow
2. Light-reflecting eye shadow
3. Sheer lipstick

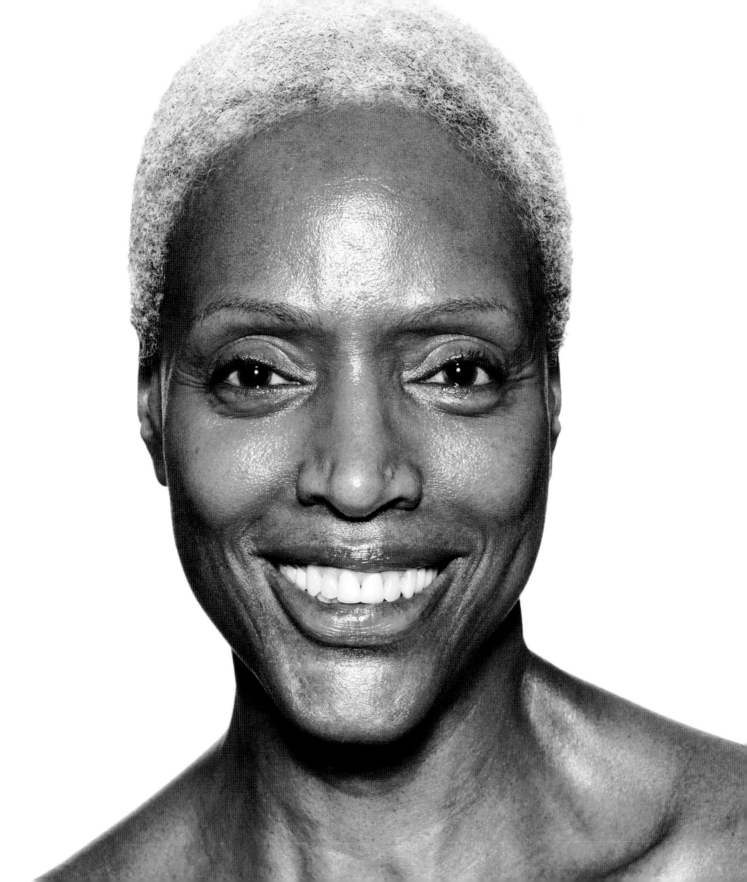

COLORFUL
COCO

Coco, 67, is a former elementary school teacher who traveled around the world as a model in the 1980s. Today, this energetic New York–based woman works at a nonprofit organization that helps high school students obtain scholarships and prepare for college.

Are there any beauty tips or tricks your family members passed on to you that you still use?

My grandmother taught me how to make a special toothpaste—a mixture of peroxide, baking soda, coconut oil, and apple cider vinegar. This also doubles as a facial cleanser. I use witch hazel as a toner and coconut oil as a nighttime moisturizer. I also use coconut oil on my body and hair.

How has the meaning of beauty changed for you through the years?

The meaning of beauty has not changed for me. I was taught that beauty has nothing to do with the color of your skin or the texture of your hair. Rather, it is the intent of a person's heart.

What are your daily beauty routines?

In the morning I cleanse my face, then use a toner. Then I apply an eye cream and an SPF-30 facial moisturizer. For the evening I go through the same routine except I use a night cream. Twice a week I exfoliate my skin and use a clay mask, because I have combination skin.

Do you have any beauty wisdom for the next generation?

Drink lots of water, get lots of sleep, surround yourself with people who love you, and remember to dance and laugh!

What makes you feel beautiful?

Being healthy makes me feel beautiful. Being able to walk tall and represent my race, my family, and my God makes me feel beautiful. I also feel beautiful when I can help other people.

What is your motto for life?

I can do all things through Christ who strengthens me (Philippians 4:13).

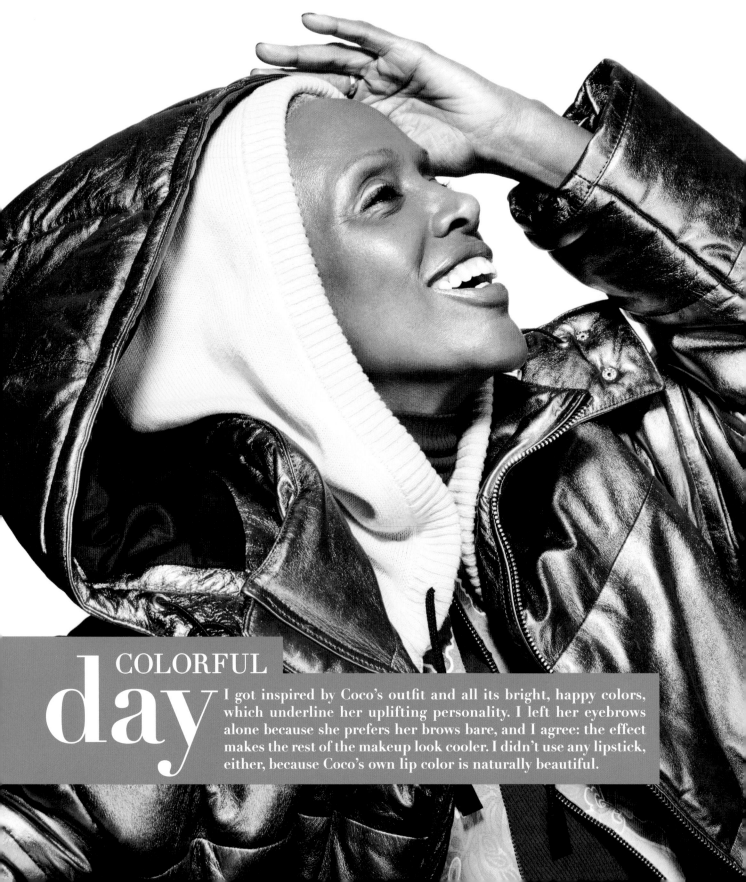

COLORFUL
day

I got inspired by Coco's outfit and all its bright, happy colors, which underline her uplifting personality. I left her eyebrows alone because she prefers her brows bare, and I agree: the effect makes the rest of the makeup look cooler. I didn't use any lipstick, either, because Coco's own lip color is naturally beautiful.

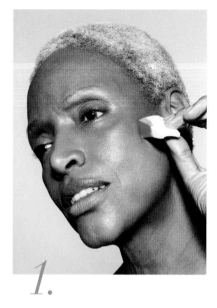

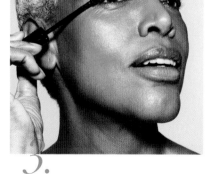

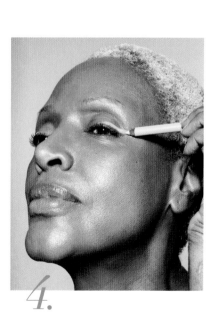

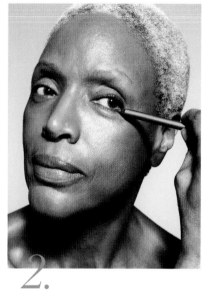

1.

2.

3.

4.

1. Coco applied bright coral cream blush with a latex-free triangle-shaped sponge for a sheer and dewy look.

2. I chose a blue-green waterproof pencil liner to bring out her eyes. She applied it on the upper lash line as well as on the waterline.

3. Next, Coco applied black waterproof mascara.

4. Then she applied a light turquoise waterproof pencil liner on top of the blue-green for a double-liner effect.

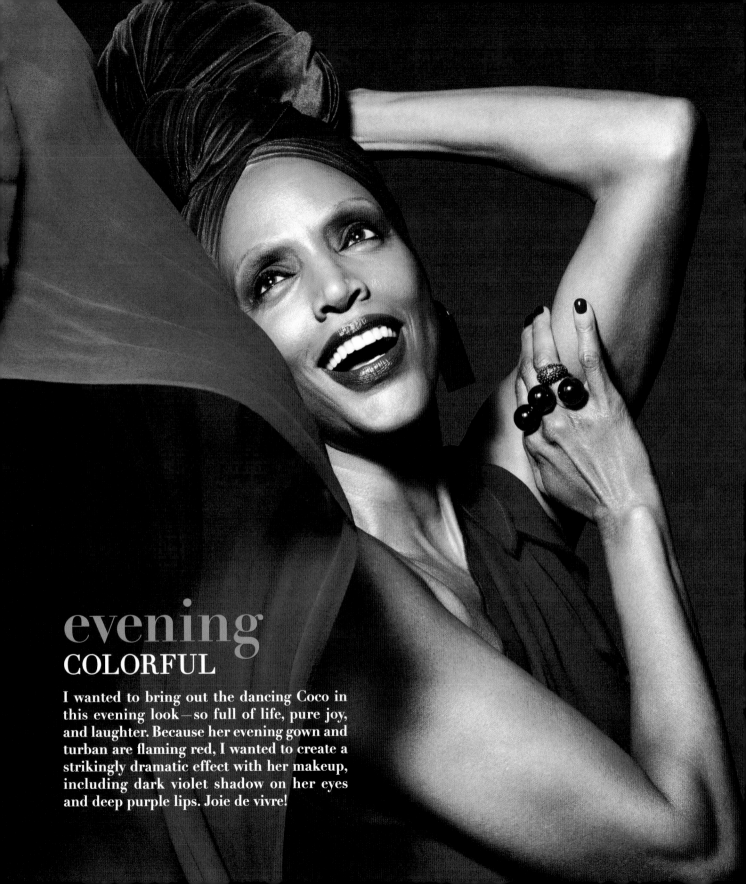

evening
COLORFUL

I wanted to bring out the dancing Coco in this evening look—so full of life, pure joy, and laughter. Because her evening gown and turban are flaming red, I wanted to create a strikingly dramatic effect with her makeup, including dark violet shadow on her eyes and deep purple lips. Joie de vivre!

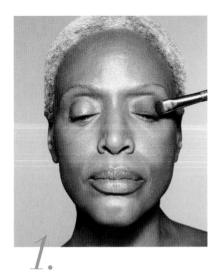

1.

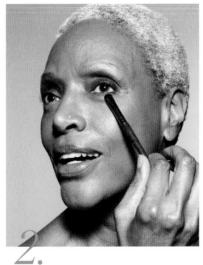

2.

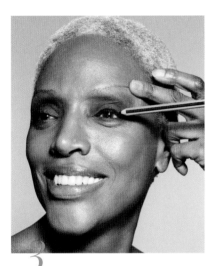

3.

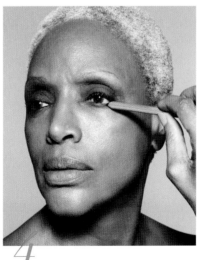

4.

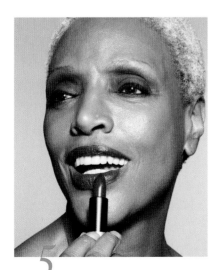

5.

1. Coco applied purple matte eye shadow on her entire lid up to the crease with a full round brush (#8 on page 25) and blended it well.

2. She used a smaller brush (#7) to apply and blend the same color on her lower lash line.

3. Then she applied black pencil liner on her upper lash line to give depth to her eyes.

4. Coco also applied black liner on her waterline.

5. Finally she applied a creamy deep purple lipstick straight from the tube all over her lips. She pressed her lips together and moved them back and forth so the lipstick settled evenly.

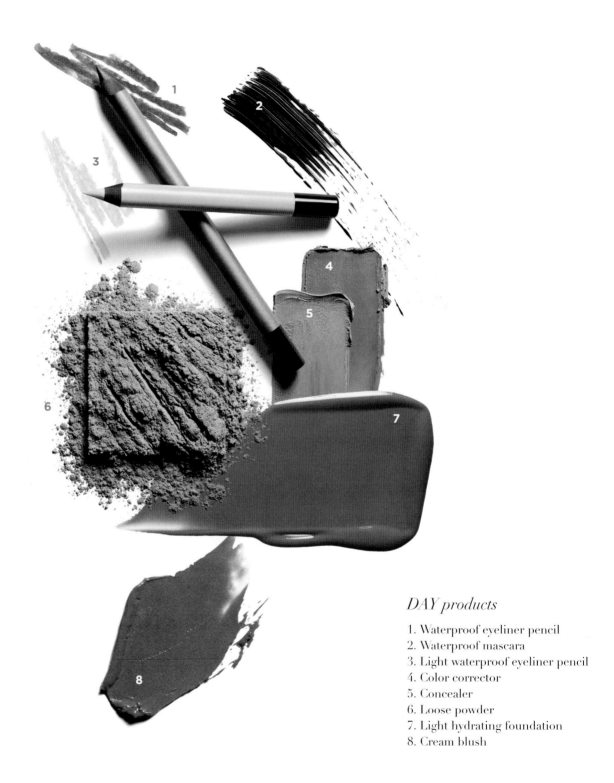

DAY products

1. Waterproof eyeliner pencil
2. Waterproof mascara
3. Light waterproof eyeliner pencil
4. Color corrector
5. Concealer
6. Loose powder
7. Light hydrating foundation
8. Cream blush

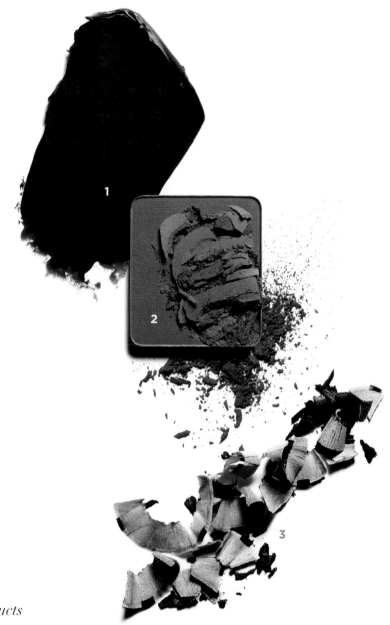

EVENING products

1. Creamy lipstick
2. Matte eye shadow
3. Eyeliner pencil

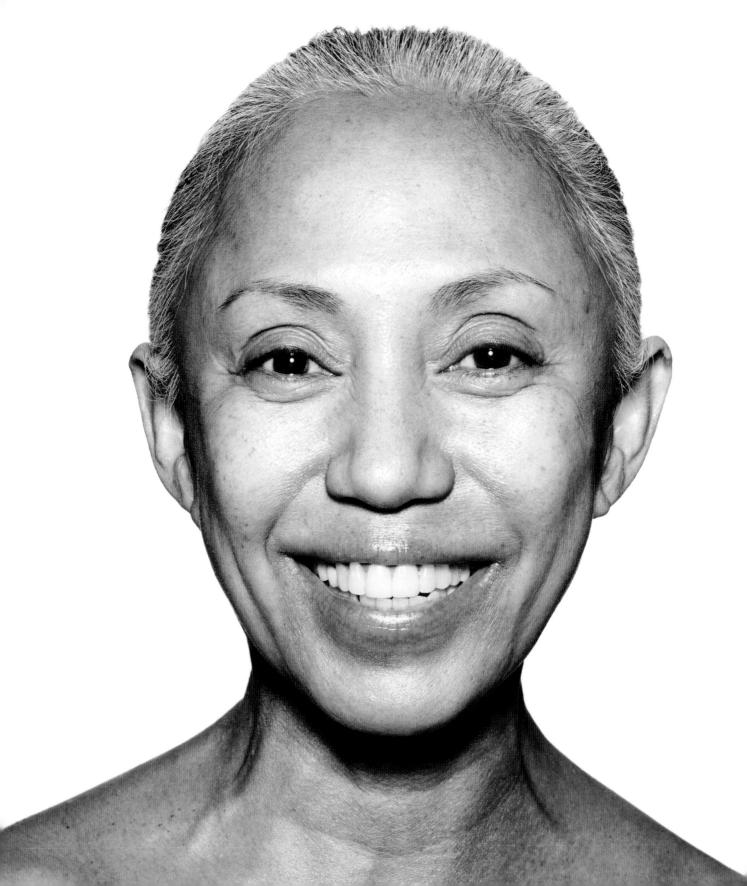

PERFORMANCE ARTIST ELIZABETH

Elizabeth, 61, was born in Manila and later became the youngest member of the Ballet Philippines. After studying dance in New York City, she performed with the Metropolitan Opera Ballet and the Alvin Ailey American Dance Theater and danced on Broadway in The King and I *as Eliza. In 1997, she was cited by* Avenue *magazine as one of the five hundred most influential Asian Americans. Today, she creates choreography for regional theaters and teaches dance and performance to Actors Studio Drama School students at the Ailey School.*

Are there any beauty tips or tricks your family members passed on to you that you still use?

There were three women in my life whom I grew up with and learned from. My grandmother, mother, and aunt were an integral part of my introduction to beauty. What I saw each of them do informed me as I grew up. My grandmother never used soap on her face. My mother, it was said, had a virgin's face because her eyes, mouth, and nose were all the same width. She used Vaseline on her eyelashes to get some glimmer on them, and she rubbed olive oil on her body and face to moisturize her skin. My aunt always made sure her eyebrows were perfectly arched, shaped, and penciled.

How has the meaning of beauty changed for you through the years?

I once thought, while growing up in the Philippines, that I was an ugly duckling, particularly because I was the only female child living with three elegant women. There was a notion that lighter skin was better, so my grandmother would bleach my skin on the weekends with bleaching creams, which I hated. I didn't understand it. My grandmother never left the house without an umbrella.

I love the sun. For many years, the dark-skin-versus-light-skin issue was confusing to me, and it was not until I came to New York City that I realized that the issue is woven into the very fabric of society. It was when I became the only Filipina in a major dance company that I came to appreciate the many differences that distinguish me. Those differences made me more, not less.

What are your daily beauty routines?

They are very simple. I use a nondrying face cleanser (as my grandmother advised, I never wash my face with soap), a good moisturizer for my neck and face, eye cream, and of course sunblock, which I apply on top of my day cream. It also helps to have a good dermatologist. I believe as one ages, one needs less makeup, unless of course you're going to a festive event. I always make sure my eyebrows are done, though!

Do you have any beauty wisdom for the next generation?

Stress is always a big problem, and its effects show on your face. You have to find a way to relax. I have been chanting for the last thirty-seven years. It is my therapy and my therapist.

Sing out loud, even when you are off-key! I love Puccini's aria "O mio babbino caro," and I sing it loud. Also, my husband and I make sure to laugh, talk, cry, and allow ourselves to feel. He loves me very much.

Sometimes there are days when I look in the mirror and say, "Ugh." Then there are days when I say, "Wow." Cherish, enjoy, and remember those moments. And if you are lucky enough to have a partner who adores you, loves you, and supports you, then that's another feather in your cap!

What makes you feel beautiful, and what does beauty mean to you?

My home, my love, and my friends. When I look in the mirror, I don't see an ugly duckling anymore. I see a girl who became a woman and has come into her own by experiencing life's vicissitudes. I see someone who is stronger than she thinks she is, someone who has substance, and someone who continues to be a creative and compassionate person. I hope that each line and crevice on my face and body, which have come with years of life's ups and downs, have added to my beauty and character.

What is your motto for life?

A Buddhist word of wisdom: envying another's beauty will diminish your own. But when you praise beauty in others, your own beauty deepens.

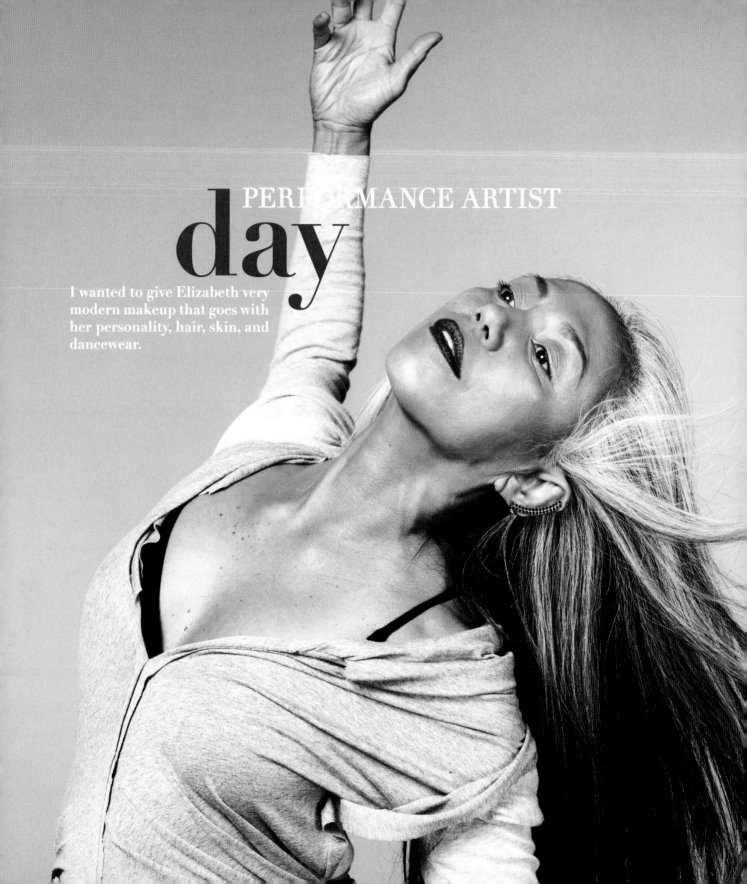

PERFORMANCE ARTIST
day

I wanted to give Elizabeth very modern makeup that goes with her personality, hair, skin, and dancewear.

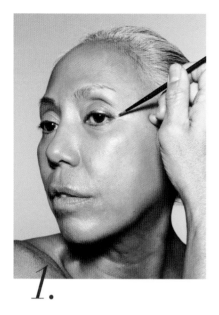

1.

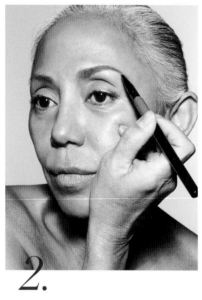

2.

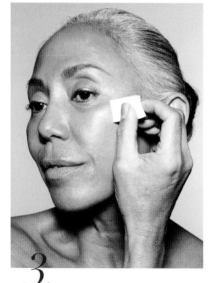

3.

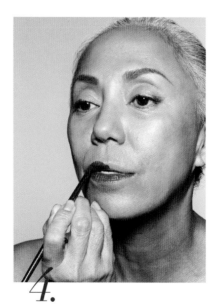

4.

1. I chose a silver waterproof eyeliner—a very simple detail—applied with an eyeliner brush (#11 on page 25) and extended a bit. When you have gray hair, a silver liner looks just fabulous. You don't need to add any other makeup on the eyelids.

2. Elizabeth fills in her brows every day. I chose an eyebrow pencil that is easy to use and matches her hair color perfectly.

3. Elizabeth used a latex-free triangle-shaped sponge to apply golden highlighter to her cheeks, which accentuates her beautiful high cheekbones.

4. Dark purple cream lipstick looks great on Elizabeth's yellow-golden skin. Cream lipstick contains more wax than sheer lipstick, so the texture feels thicker. It also stays on longer than sheer lipstick, which contains more oil. Elizabeth applied it with a lip brush (#12), then pressed her lips together to allow the color to blend naturally.

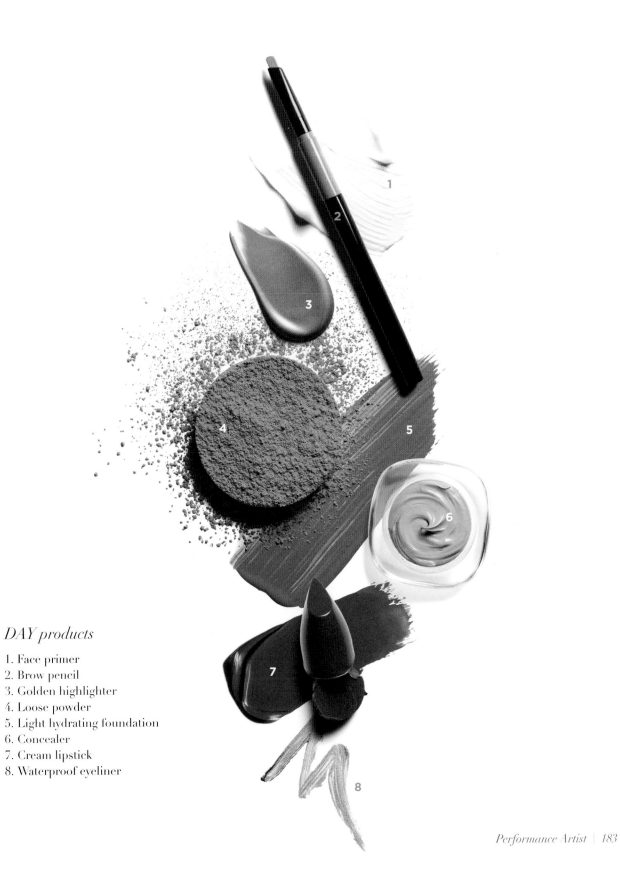

DAY products

1. Face primer
2. Brow pencil
3. Golden highlighter
4. Loose powder
5. Light hydrating foundation
6. Concealer
7. Cream lipstick
8. Waterproof eyeliner

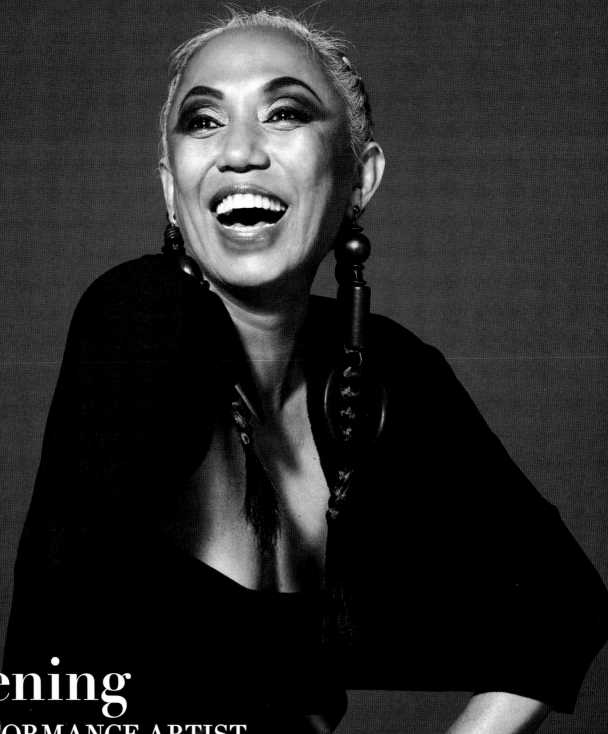

evening
PERFORMANCE ARTIST

For special events, Elizabeth loves to bring out her big, beautiful eyes. I wanted to give her black-and-silver eye makeup and keep the rest of her face very natural. It is important to use an eyelid primer for evening makeup like this so the shadows won't crease on the lids.

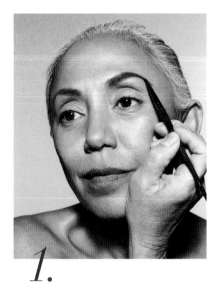

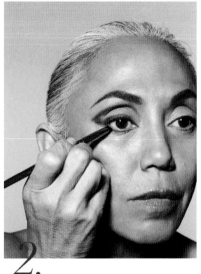

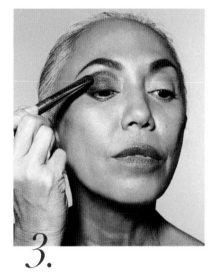

1. First I wanted to darken Elizabeth's eyebrows with a dark ash-gray color, which she applied with a brow brush (#10 on page 25).

2. This makeup is all about extending the eyes, almost creating a cat's eye. I chose a semimatte eye shadow that reflects a bit of light—beautiful for evening. Elizabeth used a small round brush (#7) to line her eyes with black shadow, applying it to the roots of her upper lash line. She extended the line over the outer corner of the eye and connected it with a line drawn on the crease of the eyelid. She did the same with her lower lash line.

3. Then she filled the space between the lines with black shadow, leaving the inner corners open.

4. Elizabeth applied silver eye shadow to the inner corners of her eyes and blended it toward the outer corner, so the silver ran over into the black. She also added silver shadow on the bottom lash line as a highlighter.

5. Next she applied black eyeliner pencil on the roots of the lashes as well on the upper and lower waterlines.

6. Using a blush brush (#6), she applied matte bronzer just below the cheekbones and blended it well, which gives a beautiful contour.

7. For a natural look, Elizabeth used her index finger to tap sheer lipstick onto her lips.

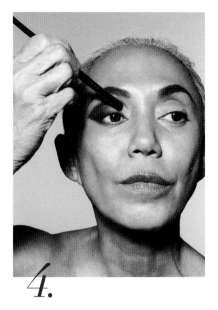

4.

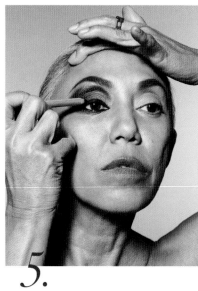

5.

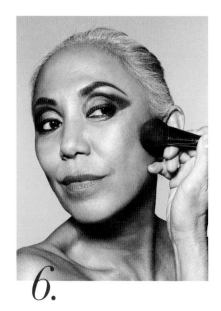

6.

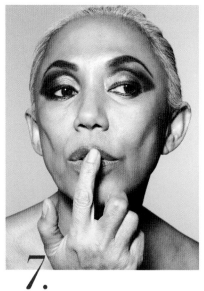

7.

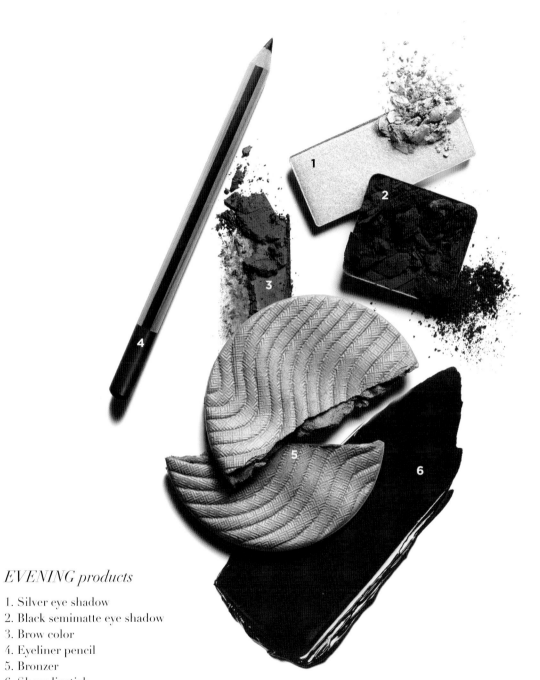

EVENING products

1. Silver eye shadow
2. Black semimatte eye shadow
3. Brow color
4. Eyeliner pencil
5. Bronzer
6. Sheer lipstick

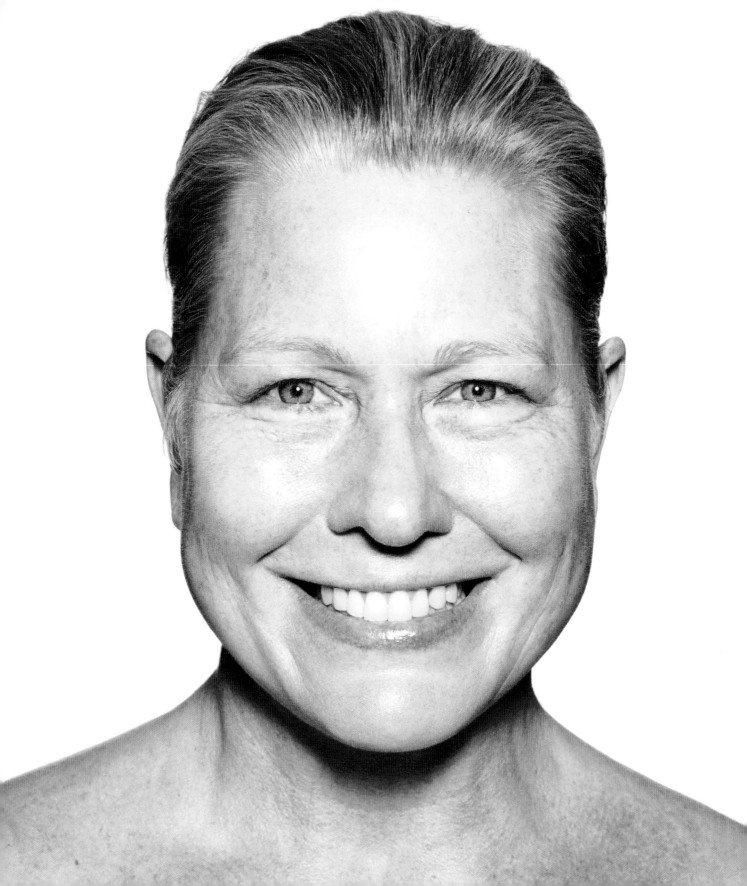

56

CLASSIC GLAMOUR
EMME

Plus-size model Emme, 56, has been breaking barriers in the fashion and beauty industry ever since she stepped into the spotlight. In 1994, she became the first full-figured model People *magazine chose for its "50 Most Beautiful People" issue. She was chosen again in 1999.*

Are there any beauty tips or tricks your family members passed on to you that you still use?

One of my favorite memories is watching my mother perform one of her beauty rituals before she went on dates with our dad. She applied whipped egg whites onto her freshly washed face. I'd try to make her smile and crack this natural mask, which in minutes got hard around her eyes, mouth, and neck. She swore the mask took away fine lines and made her skin look radiant. Now I use the egg-white mask and rub the underside of pineapple skin on my face. I leave the juice, with all its enzymes, in place for thirty minutes. It tightens and invigorates my skin! Love!

How has the meaning of beauty changed for you through the years?

As I push forward decade after decade, I see the need to reevaluate what beauty means for me. When I was younger, "beauty" was fed to me via media images. Now, in midlife, I own my beauty, no longer being told what beauty looks like. I have opened up my own aperture: what beauty looks like to me is how a person laughs, smiles, stands in her own grace, and owns the space she inhabits.

I no longer follow the one-dimensional ideal I once thought beauty was. The beauty of nature brings me to my knees. I have been able to see it in many different forms and people than ever before.

What are your daily beauty routines?

I use a cleansing oil to wash my makeup off every night, followed by eye makeup remover, a face serum, and night cream. In the winter, before and after skiing or going on long snowshoeing treks, I put a thick layer of coconut oil on my skin, which seems to act as a barrier to the harsh cold weather. I dry-brush my body and face every two weeks.

Do you have any beauty wisdom for the next generation?

Eat clean: low sugar, low dairy, no sodas or highly processed foods, and absolutely no smoking cigarettes or e-cigarettes! Drink water: more times than not, women are dehydrated, which can cause wrinkles.

What makes you feel beautiful, and what does beauty mean to you?

I feel the most beautiful after sex. You did ask! Beauty in my everyday life could be the feel of a luxurious fabric on my skin, the way a pair of well-fitting jeans hugs my curves, a gloss that makes my lips look succulent, the way on certain days my hair falls just right, or a perfect cup of coffee drunk while watching the sun rise.

What is your motto for life?

As Tony Robbins said, we change when the pain of not changing is greater than the change itself. The more I resist the most consistent thing in life, change, the more I suffer. So my goal is to notice the signs that change is needed and go with the flow. At the end of the day, why suffer? Go with the flow. Long-held beliefs that don't serve you are meant to be reevaluated.

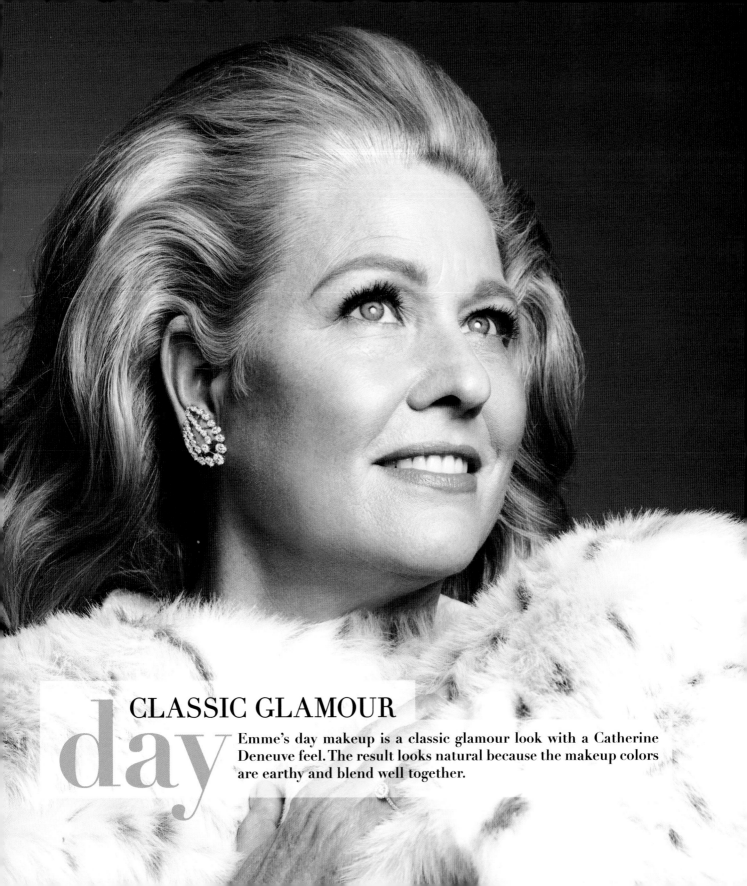

CLASSIC GLAMOUR

day

Emme's day makeup is a classic glamour look with a Catherine Deneuve feel. The result looks natural because the makeup colors are earthy and blend well together.

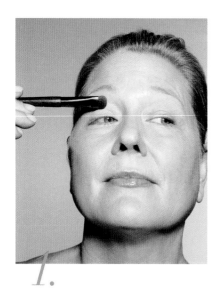

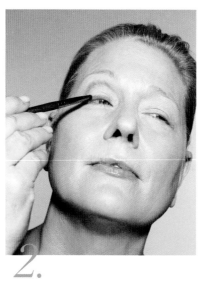

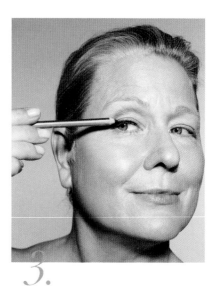

1. Emme started by applying light matte eye shadow on her entire eyelid with a large round brush (#8 on page 25). This light base color opens the eyes.

2. She used a classic eye makeup technique: applying dark matte eye shadow on the roots of the lashes and the crease with a small round brush (#7). This gives depth and dimension to the eyes. It also makes them look bigger.

3. She applied dark brown eyeliner to the roots of the lashes. The liner really brings the eyes to life. Every woman should own a pencil liner. And, of course, she applied a coat of mascara.

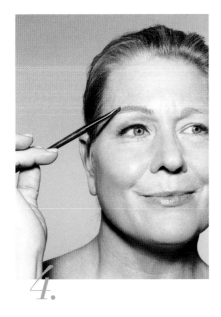

4.

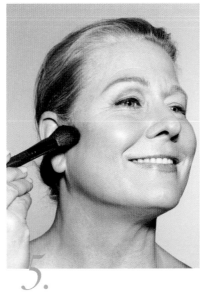

5.

6.

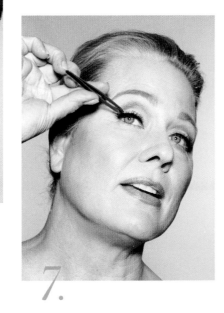

7.

4. For a classic glamour look, the brows must be perfect. After powdering her brows, Emme fills them in with taupe brow pencil.

5. A matte bronzer was used as to contour Emme's face, giving definition to her cheekbones and warmth to her face. She applied the color just below the cheekbones with a blush brush (#6).

6. Emme lined her lips with a peach liner pencil and applied the same color lipstick on top. This color is perfect for light skin tones.

7. A short strip of false eyelashes creates fullness but doesn't make Emme look too made-up. She applied a thin coat of glue to the base of the strip, waited twenty seconds for the glue to get tacky, then carefully applied the lashes with tweezers as close to the lash line as possible.

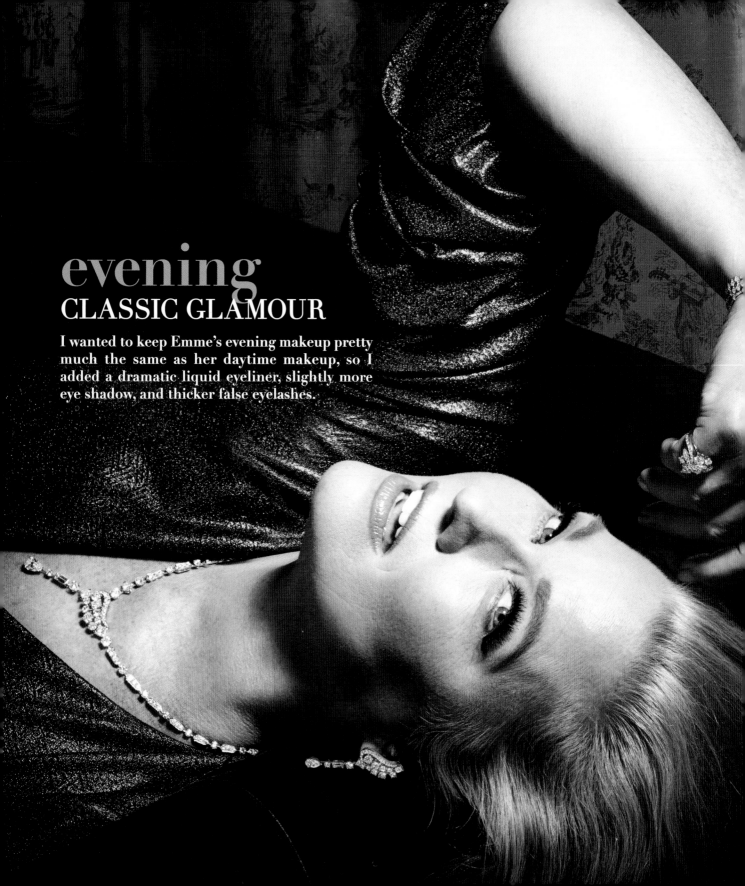

evening
CLASSIC GLAMOUR

I wanted to keep Emme's evening makeup pretty much the same as her daytime makeup, so I added a dramatic liquid eyeliner, slightly more eye shadow, and thicker false eyelashes.

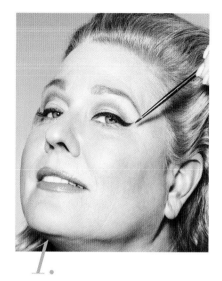

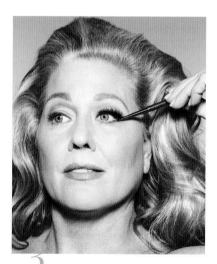

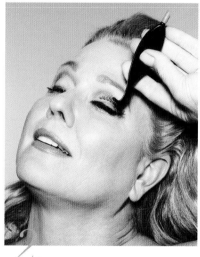

1. When adding drama to the eyes, I like to work with gel liners because they glide on more easily than liquid liners. Emme thickened the line with an eyeliner brush (#11 on page 25) and extended the ends into "wings."

2. This time Emme applied a fuller strip of false eyelashes. As she did for her day look, she applied a thin coat of glue to the base of the strip, waited twenty seconds for the glue to get tacky, then carefully put them as close to the lash line as possible. Here she used an applicator.

3. Using an eyeliner brush, she added more brown eye shadow to the outer corners of her bottom lash lines to open the eyes.

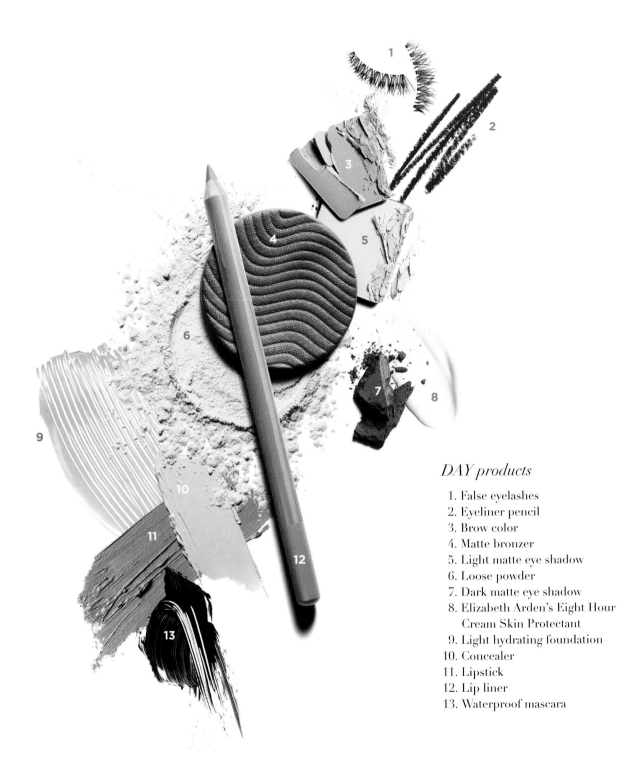

DAY products

1. False eyelashes
2. Eyeliner pencil
3. Brow color
4. Matte bronzer
5. Light matte eye shadow
6. Loose powder
7. Dark matte eye shadow
8. Elizabeth Arden's Eight Hour
   Cream Skin Protectant
9. Light hydrating foundation
10. Concealer
11. Lipstick
12. Lip liner
13. Waterproof mascara

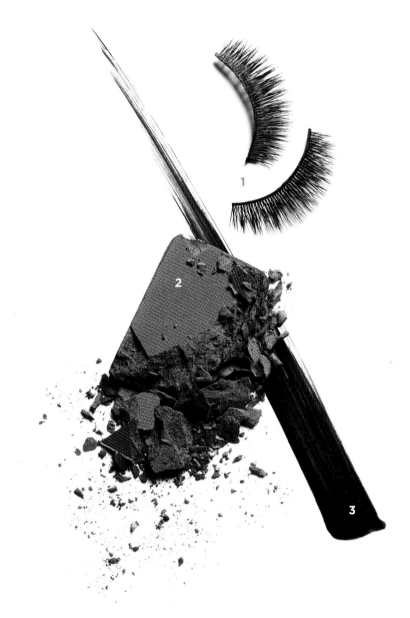

EVENING products

1. False eyelashes
2. Matte eye shadow
3. Gel liner

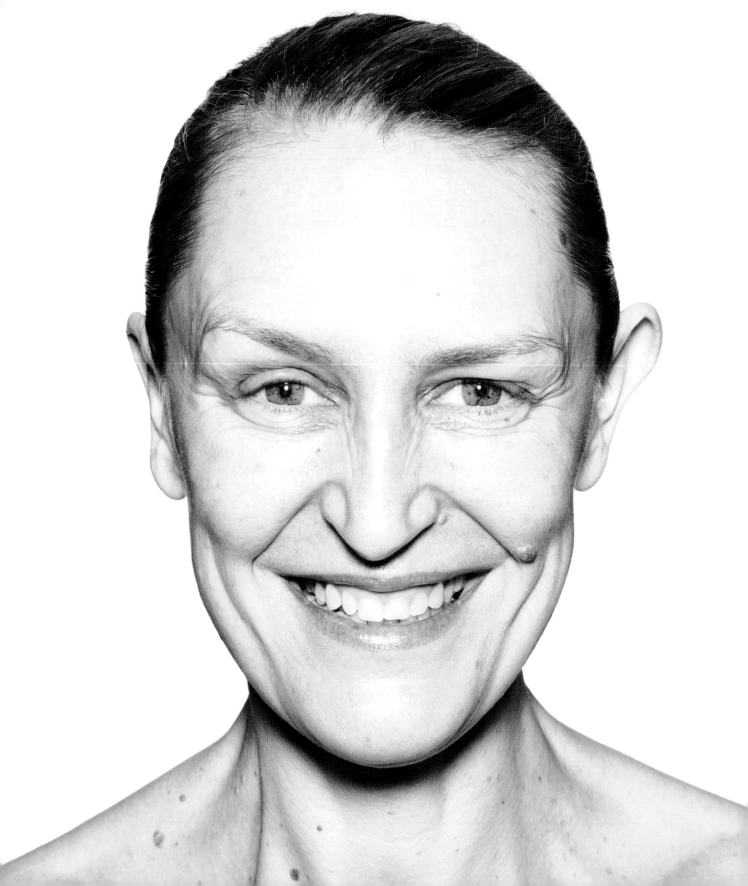

MODERN CHIC
SABINE

A world traveler, Sabine, 54, is a wardrobe stylist and the fashion editor of A Green Beauty *magazine. She likes to describe herself and her style as* Je ne sais quoi, *meaning she can't be explained. Sabine treats her skin with natural ingredients from her own kitchen, and she believes in organic food and meditation.*

Are there any beauty tips or tricks your family members passed on to you that you still use?

Not particularly—just the idea that less is more.

How has the meaning of beauty changed for you through the years?

It has simplified. I went from striving for made-up beauty to wanting to be natural.

What are your daily beauty routines?

In the morning, I massage almond oil onto my face before taking a shower and rubbing it off with a cloth. Then I massage a few drops of another face oil into my skin. I always wear concealer, nude eye shadow, and red lipstick—that's the Frenchwoman in me. In the evening, I remove my makeup with a damp cotton ball moistened with sesame oil, then I spray rose-water toner on my face and follow with face oil.

In the winter I treat myself to an egg-yolk-and-honey mask, and in the summer I switch to a lemon-and-honey mask.

Do you have any beauty wisdom for the next generation?

Take the time to eat well and meditate.

What makes you feel beautiful, and what does beauty mean to you?

Red lipstick makes me feel beautiful. Beauty is finding a balance—one that helps you navigate the hills and valleys of the day with grace. It's also the ability to put a smile on someone else's face.

What is your motto for life?

In truth, a quotation from Carl Sagan: "I don't know where I'm going, but I'm on my way."

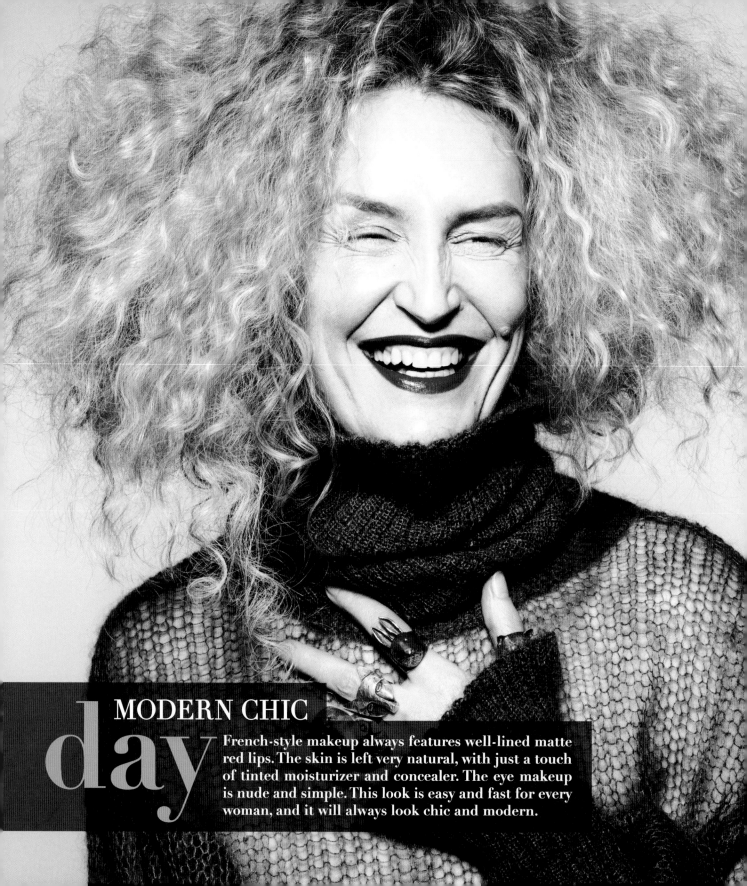

MODERN CHIC
day

French-style makeup always features well-lined matte red lips. The skin is left very natural, with just a touch of tinted moisturizer and concealer. The eye makeup is nude and simple. This look is easy and fast for every woman, and it will always look chic and modern.

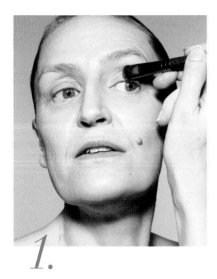

1.

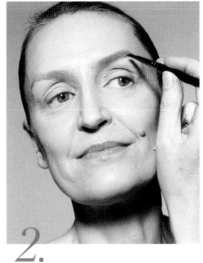

2.

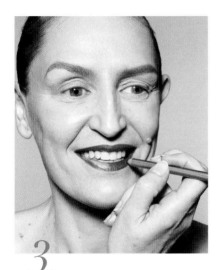

3.

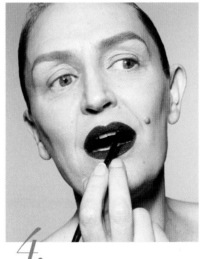

4.

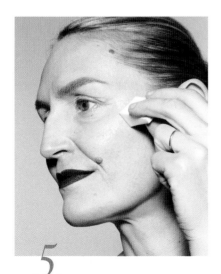

5.

1. First Sabine swept a light sand-color matte eye shadow on the lids using a large round brush (#8 on page 25).

2. Sabine used an eyebrow brush (#10) to fill in her brows with taupe-colored powder. Then she brushed them with brow gel.

3. She then lined and filled her lips with a red lip pencil. This technique makes the lipstick last.

4. Sabine used a lip brush (#12) to apply the perfect red cream lipstick on top of the lip liner.

5. Instead of blush, I chose a gold-based highlighter for her cheeks that works beautifully with matte lips.

evening
MODERN CHIC

While Sabine's hair was pulled back, her beautiful profile inspired me to give her a slightly androgynous look, with darker brows and light smoky eyes. I used no lipstick or mascara.

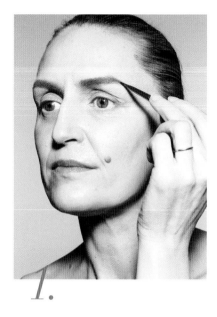

1.

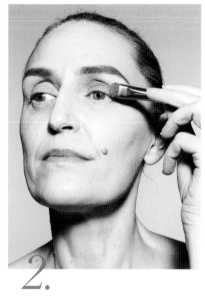

2.

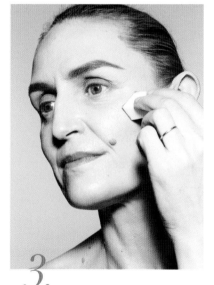

3.

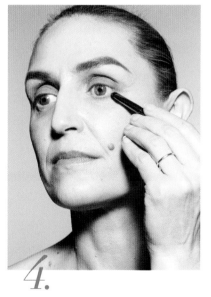

4.

1. I wanted Sabine's brows to have a more masculine vibe, so I chose a brow color slightly darker than her own natural brows. She filled them in with a brow brush (#10 on page 25). Then we sprayed a little hair spray onto the brush and brushed the brows to keep them in place. The spray is a great substitute for brow gel.

2. Taupe is a good color if you want a lightly smoky eye, especially on Sabine's fair skin. She used a large round brush (#8) to apply the shadow on the entire lid up to the crease, then blended it well.

3. Sabine then added a bit of light-pink cream blush to warm up her face.

4. A touch of the eye shadow on the lower lash line made Sabine's eyes bigger and more open.

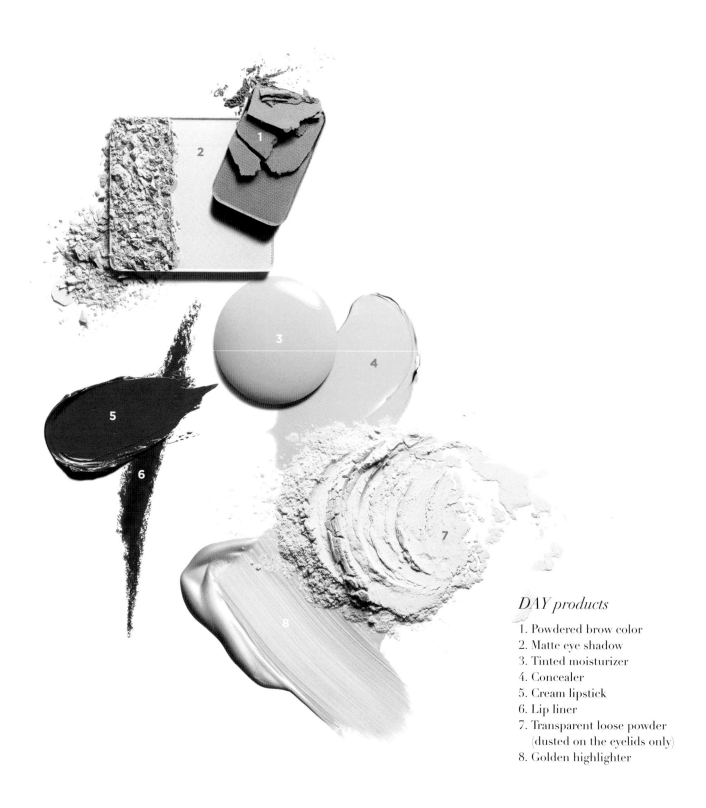

DAY products

1. Powdered brow color
2. Matte eye shadow
3. Tinted moisturizer
4. Concealer
5. Cream lipstick
6. Lip liner
7. Transparent loose powder
   (dusted on the eyelids only)
8. Golden highlighter

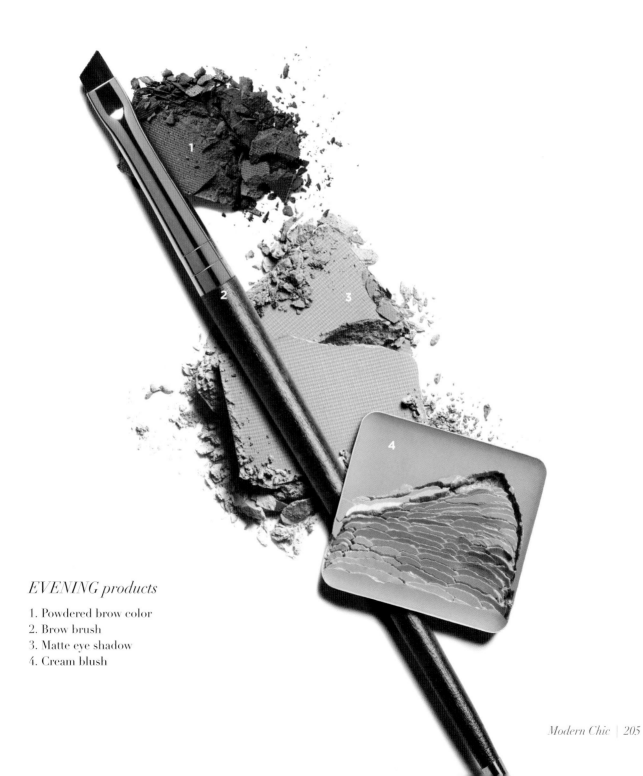

EVENING products

1. Powdered brow color
2. Brow brush
3. Matte eye shadow
4. Cream blush

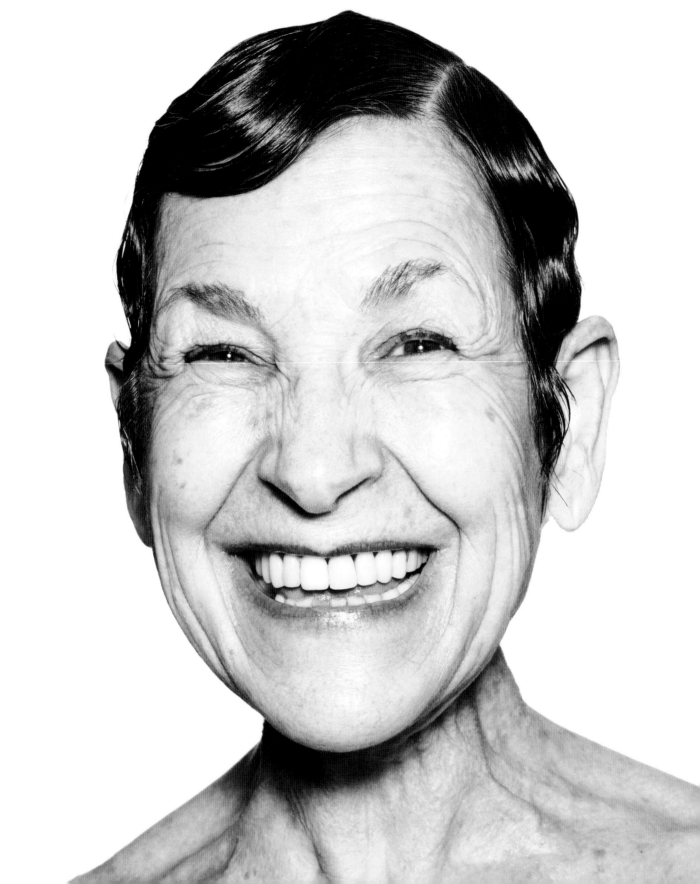

STYLE ICON
TZIPORAH

Born in Israel to Hungarian parents, New York City resident Tziporah, 70, is the irrepressible voice and champion of women who dare to dress. She has spent a lifetime collecting remarkable antique clothing, hats, and accessories. She has been featured in publications such as Vogue, New York *magazine, and the* New York Times. *She modeled for couture houses such as Lanvin, was a muse for the late photographer Bill Cunningham, and runs a style seminar called the Art of Dressing.*

Are there any beauty tips or tricks your family members passed on to you that you still use?

My mother was Hungarian, and like all Hungarian women, she had flawless skin. She believed in facials, and starting when I was very young, she took me for facials on a regular basis. She taught me the importance of taking good care of my skin by eating fresh fruits and vegetables and keeping it all quite simple.

How has the meaning of beauty changed for you through the years?

I still thrive on beauty. It enriches my life. It has to be beautiful around me or I wilt. Beauty lifts my spirit. I seek it and find it everywhere. Better still, beauty finds me. And everywhere I look, there is beauty.

What are your daily beauty routines?

I keep it simple. Wash, tone, moisturize. Some eye shadow and mascara, a light foundation, and I always put on red lipstick.

Do you have any beauty wisdom for the next generation?

Allow yourself to age gracefully. There is nothing more beautiful than a woman whose face shows the markers of time.

What makes you feel beautiful, and what does beauty mean to you?

I feel beautiful when I am comfortable in my body, when I am wearing clothes that sing to me and turn me on, and when I am sharing a good laugh with a friend. Beauty is the flowers on the table, the fresh fruit in the crystal bowl, a sunrise, a sunset, and the perfect shoes.

What is your motto for life?

Since I am writing this from Costa Rica, *pura vida*!

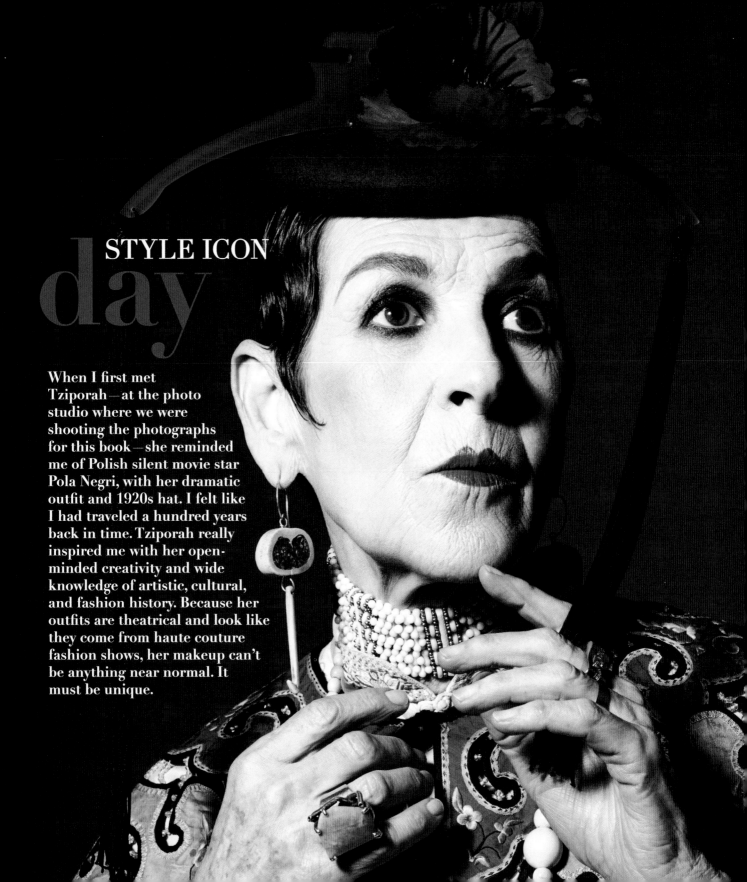

STYLE ICON
day

When I first met Tziporah—at the photo studio where we were shooting the photographs for this book—she reminded me of Polish silent movie star Pola Negri, with her dramatic outfit and 1920s hat. I felt like I had traveled a hundred years back in time. Tziporah really inspired me with her open-minded creativity and wide knowledge of artistic, cultural, and fashion history. Because her outfits are theatrical and look like they come from haute couture fashion shows, her makeup can't be anything near normal. It must be unique.

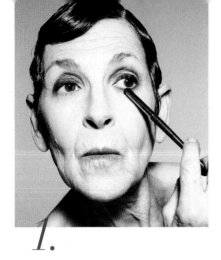

1.

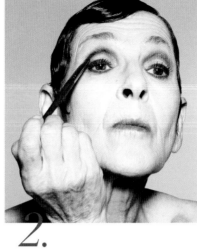

2.

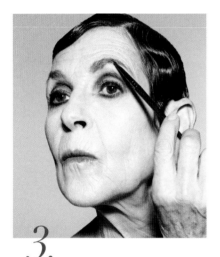

3.

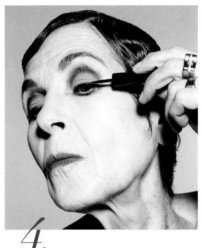

4.

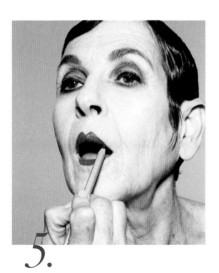

5.

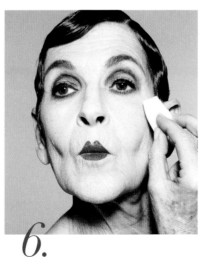

6.

1. Tziporah first applied a dark gray matte eye shadow—a kind of thick powdered liner—on her upper lash line. Then, using a small round brush (#7 on page 25), she applied it to the crease of her eyelids and the lower lash line.

2. Black matte eye shadow was applied on top of the gray to create more dimension.

3. Tziporah's eyebrows grow naturally in a round shape. Using a brow brush (#10), she darkened them a little by filling them in with a warm brown.

4. She then applied black liquid liner to her upper lash lines. She also added a lot of mascara.

5. Tziporah covered her lips completely with foundation, then drew a Cupid's bow shape on her upper lip with red lip pencil. She filled in her lips with the color.

6. Then Tziporah applied pink cream blush to the apples of her cheeks.

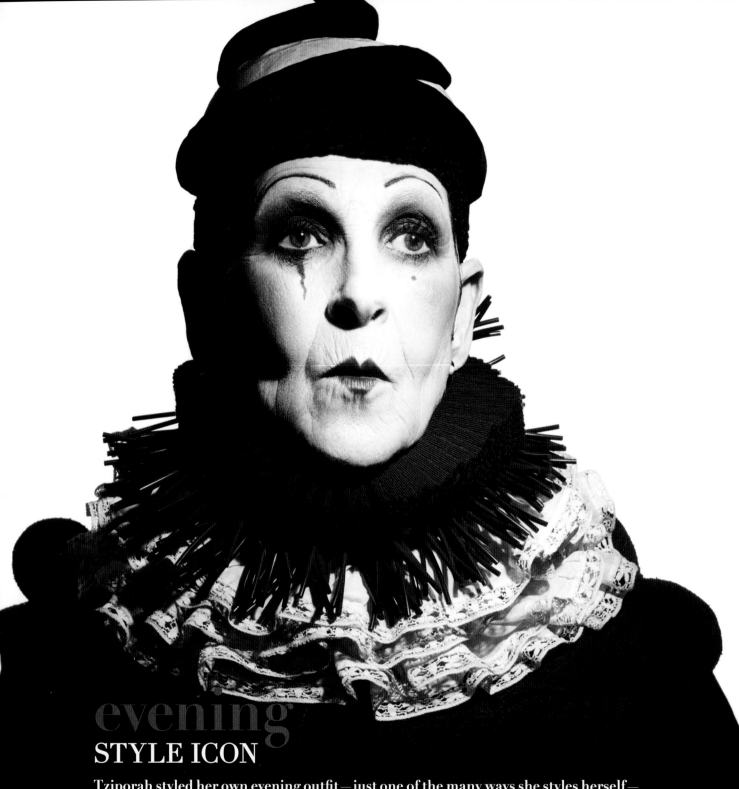

evening
STYLE ICON

Tziporah styled her own evening outfit—just one of the many ways she styles herself—and the outcome is theatrical, funny, and dramatic. She loves clowns, so I imagined her as a 1920s stage diva who's ready for a big premiere party!

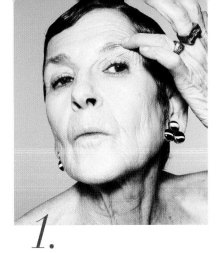

1.

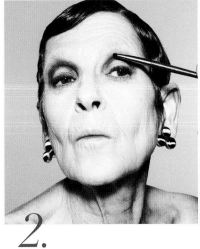

2.

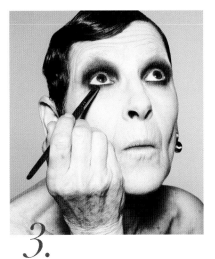

3.

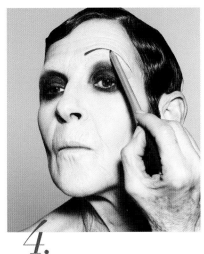

4.

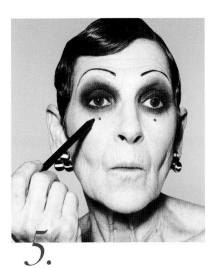

5.

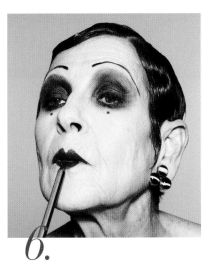

6.

1. First we hid Tziporah's brows, because in the 1920s, brows were thinner and rounder than her natural brows. She covered her eyebrows with paper glue, then applied concealer and loose powder so they were less visible.

2. Then she used a small round brush (#7 on page 25) to apply burgundy matte eye shadow first on the lash line and then on the crease of her eyelids. We also used the burgundy eye shadow as blush on her cheeks.

3. Next, she applied black eye shadow on the entire lid as well as on the lower lash line to create a dramatic, smoky style.

4. New brows were drawn with a brown pencil above Tziporah's hidden brows. She deepened the color with liquid black eyeliner.

5. She added two beauty marks under her eyes with a black waterproof eyeliner pencil.

6. Then Tziporah lined her lips in 1920s style with dark burgundy pencil and filled them in with the same pencil.

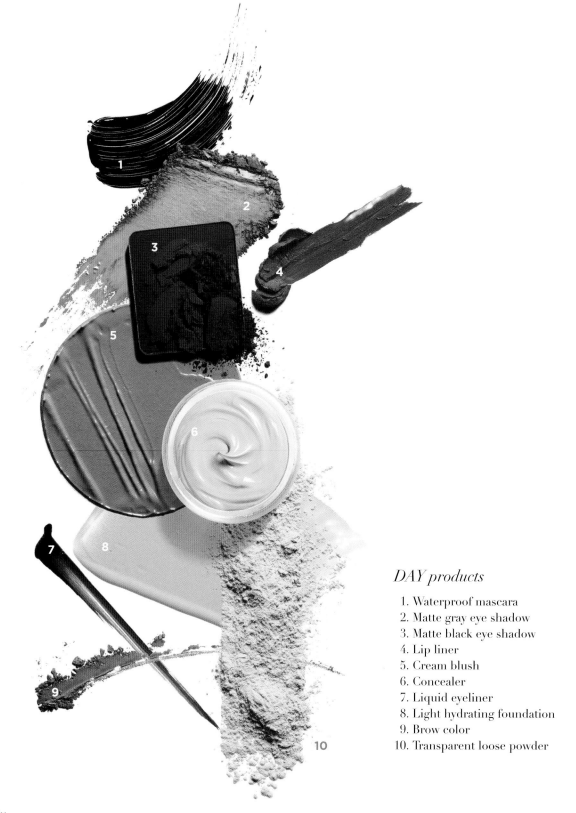

DAY products

1. Waterproof mascara
2. Matte gray eye shadow
3. Matte black eye shadow
4. Lip liner
5. Cream blush
6. Concealer
7. Liquid eyeliner
8. Light hydrating foundation
9. Brow color
10. Transparent loose powder

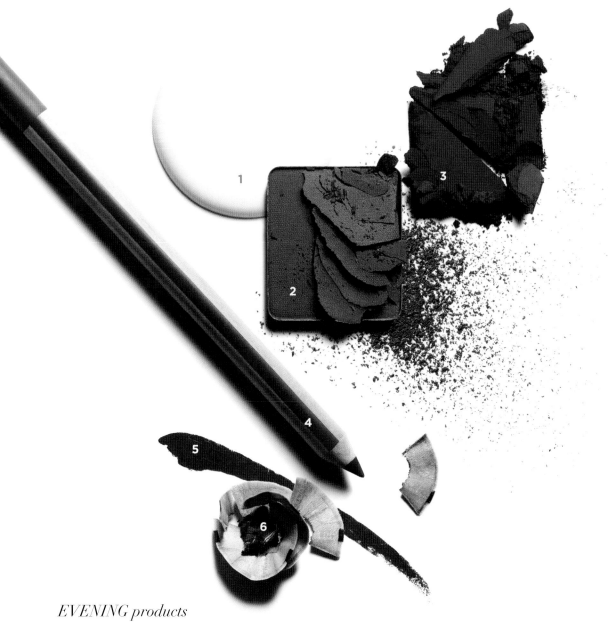

EVENING products

1. Paper glue for the eyebrows
2. Matte burgundy eye shadow
3. Matte black eye shadow
4. Lip liner
5. Liquid eyeliner
6. Eyeliner pencil

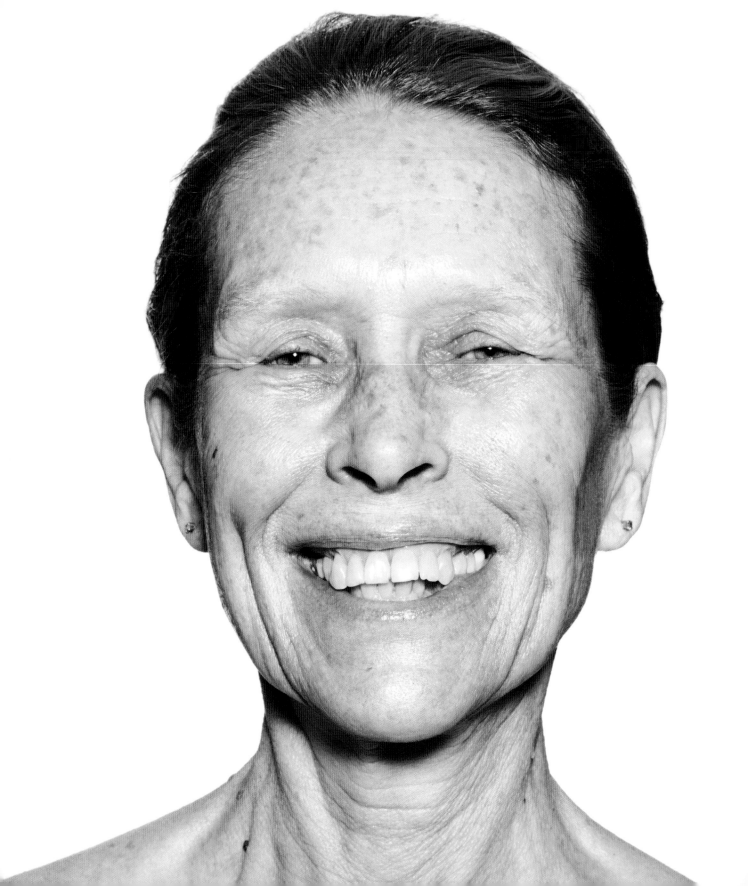

ARTIST
URSULA

I met Ursula, 63, in 2008, when she was an art director, and her style, creative direction, and work ethic inspired me. Ursula is also a multimedia artist who created the She World Archive, a collection of "lost and then found objects from the lives of women," which she has cataloged and displayed over the course of many years. Through her art she honors women's important contributions to culture.

Are there any beauty tips or tricks your family members passed on to you that you still use?

My mother and I played around with making homemade face masks out of oatmeal, honey, and other ingredients. I don't use that today, but I still prefer homemade (as opposed to store-bought) cleansers and beauty treatments.

How has the meaning of beauty changed for you through the years?

Older women often feel invisible, as if nobody looks at them. But being under constant observation can be a burden for women. I have become less concerned with how others see me. I feel more freedom to express myself in any way I want, without judgment.

What are your daily beauty routines?

Both morning and night, I apply olive oil and wash my face with Pears soap, then rinse my face twenty times in a basin of hot water. Then I apply homemade vitamin C toner (water mixed with vitamin C powder), followed by rose-hip oil at night and moisturizer with sunscreen for daytime.

Do you have any beauty wisdom for the next generation?

Don't worry too much. Beauty is destroyed by too much effort.

What makes you feel beautiful?

Feeling healthy after swimming, taking a Jacuzzi bath, and taking care of myself.

What is your motto for life?

Offer creative energy to the world, your community, and yourself.

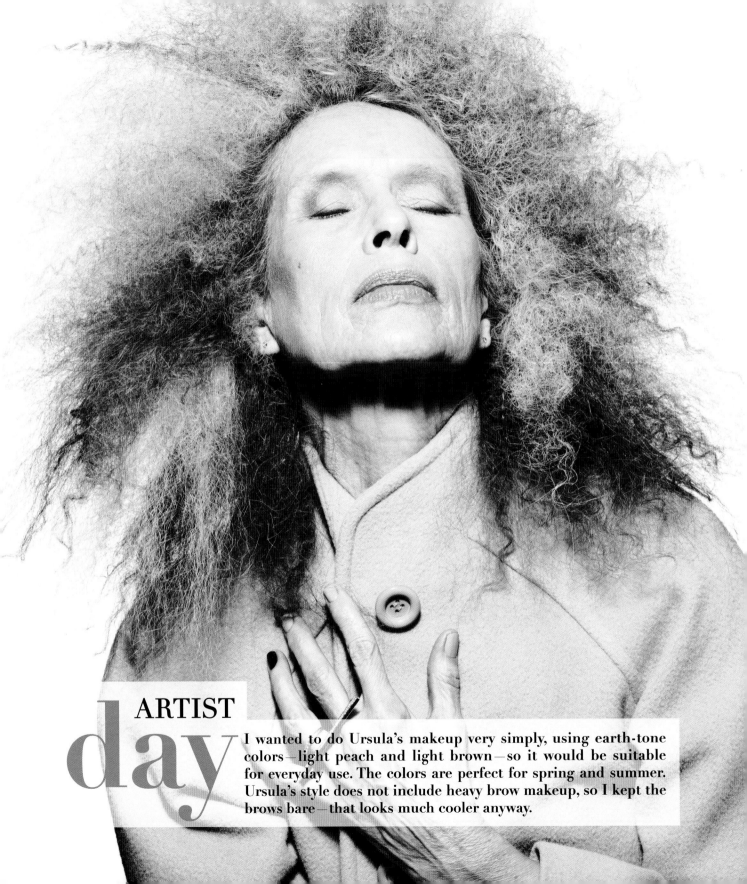

ARTIST
day

I wanted to do Ursula's makeup very simply, using earth-tone colors—light peach and light brown—so it would be suitable for everyday use. The colors are perfect for spring and summer. Ursula's style does not include heavy brow makeup, so I kept the brows bare—that looks much cooler anyway.

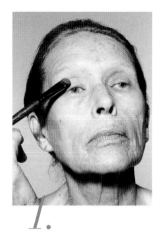

1.

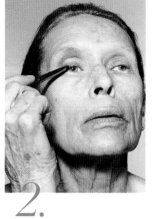

2.

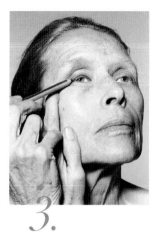

3.

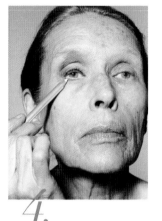

4.

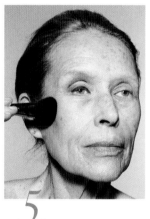

5.

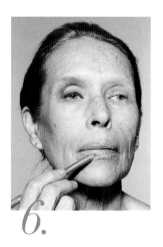

6.

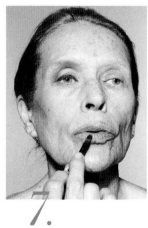

7.

4. White pencil liner on the waterline opens up the eyes and looks beautiful with earth tones.

5. A touch of peach powdered blush gives color to the cheeks. I chose powder because I wanted to keep Ursula's makeup all matte.

6. First she applied a lip primer to keep the lip liner and lipstick in place. Then she used lip liner to keep the lipstick from seeping into the fine lines around the mouth. The secret is to apply a very small amount of lipstick, just enough to cover the lips and give color. Too much lipstick will run, even if you use primer. You can always reapply your lipstick after coffee or lunch.

7. Ursula used a brush to apply her lipstick so she could control the amount of color on her lips. It is also easier to color the edges and corners of the lips this way.

1. Light matte eye shadow was applied as a base color on the lids with a large round brush (#8 on page 25). She also applied darker eye shadow on the outer corners of the crease with a small round brush (#7), then blended well so the color faded above the crease.

2. After applying transparent loose powder all over the eyelid, she applied the darker eye shadow along the lash line.

3. I chose a light brown eyeliner pencil to soften the makeup. A black liner would have looked too harsh for daytime. She also added a coat of mascara.

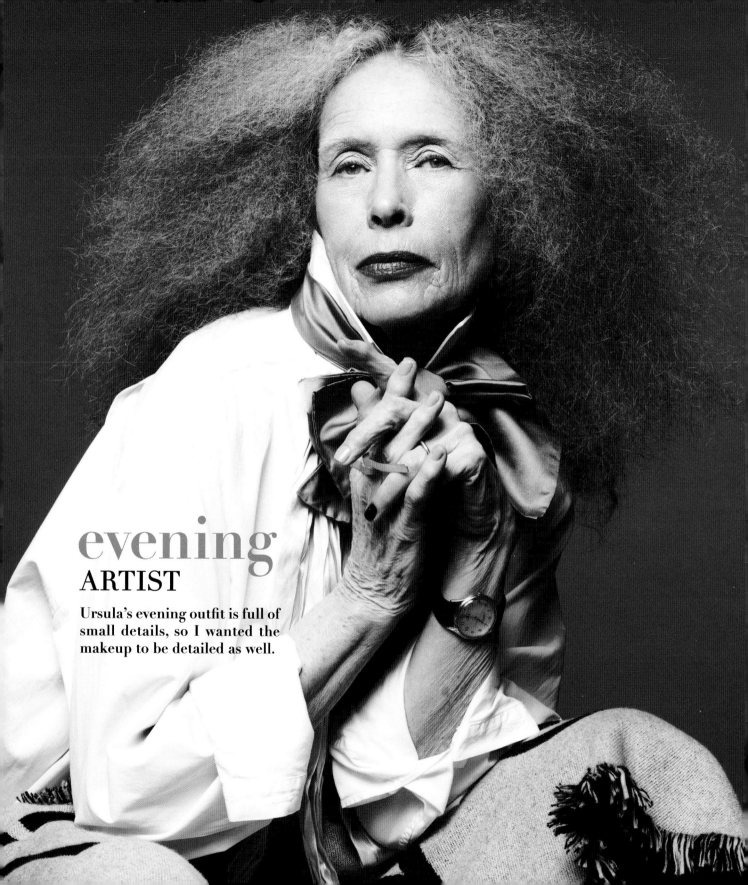

evening
ARTIST

Ursula's evening outfit is full of small details, so I wanted the makeup to be detailed as well.

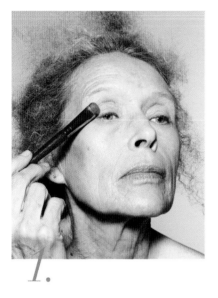

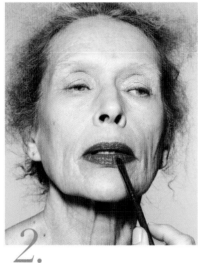

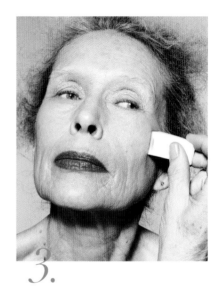

1. Light-reflecting eye shadow works the best in the evening. Ursula liked the icy blue color— she said it had 1970s flair. She applied it on her lids up to the crease with an eye shadow brush (#8 on page 25).

2. Ursula used lip primer under her lipstick so it wouldn't run into the fine lines around her mouth. She applied it with a lip brush (#12) for a soft result.

3. Light peach cream blush breaks the cool tones of the eyes and brings warmth to the cheeks.

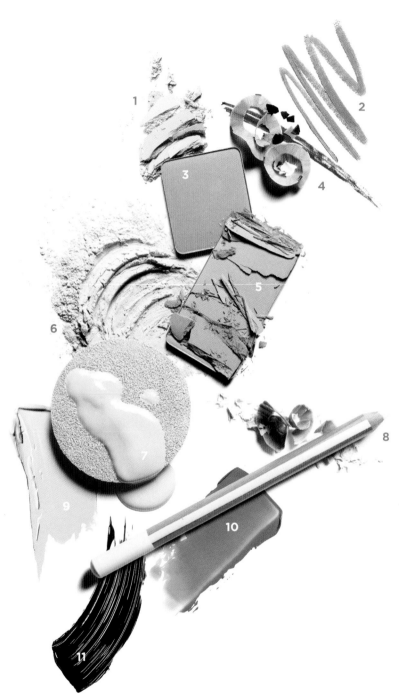

DAY products

1. Light matte eye shadow
2. Lip liner
3. Darker matte eye shadow
4. Dark eyeliner pencil
5. Powdered blush
6. Transparent loose powder
7. Light hydrating foundation
8. White eyeliner pencil
9. Color corrector (also used as a concealer)
10. Lipstick
11. Waterproof mascara

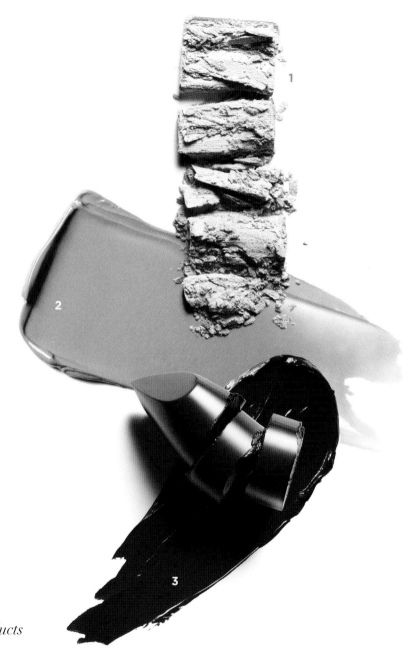

EVENING products

1. Eye shadow
2. Cream blush
3. Cream lipstick

ACKNOWLEDGMENTS

Thank you, Judith Curr, publisher at HarperOne Group, for believing in me and my vision. Thank you, Samantha Rapp, for your stunning photography and hard work. Thank you, Hilary Swanson and Aidan Mahony, for your editorial work; and thank you, Sabine Feuilloley, for your beautiful fashion styling. Thank you also to junior art director Miles Holland, Celine Kaplan PR, and all my hairstylist friends who were part of this journey: Keiko Hamaguchi, Frankie Foye, Rebecca Plymate, Carmel Bianco, Staci Child, Yukiko Tajima, Arbana Dollani, Moiz Alladina (a.k.a. Queen), Fred Van De Bunt, Frankie Payne, and Paul Fields.

Thank you especially to all the amazing, inspiring, and strong women who served as models for this book: Emme Aronson, Siobhan Bedell, Teresa Boyd, Ursula Brookbank, Jenny Brunt, Cindy Castiglioni, Shawna Christensen, Nancy Donahue, MaryAnn Elizabeth, Sabine Feuilloley, Mimi Fisher, Maarit Glocer, Ebony Haith, Zelda Josephs, Celine Kaplan, Gunilla Lindblad, Marni Malinosky, Coco Mitchell, Lana Ogilvie, Elizabeth Roxas-Dobrish, Tziporah Salamon, Tamiyo Hasegawa, Ling Tan, Pat Tracey, Allison Walton, Doreen Williams, and Karen Williams. Thank you especially, supermodel Karen Bjornson, for your support, and thank you especially, supermodel Tatjana Patitz, who flew all the way from London to shoot this project. I learned so much from each of you, and I am so thankful to have seen your inner beauty.

Thank you, Sarah Guido-Laakso, Marina Matteo at MAKE UP FOR EVER USA, Makka Elonheimo at MAKE UP FOR EVER Paris, and Caroline Greyl and Caroline Brooks at Leonor Greyl Hair.

Thank you also to Dr. Ellen Marmur and Michele S. Green, MD, and aestheticians Nachi Glick at Mist Beauty by Nachi, Danielle Gamble at Sisley Paris, and Gaby Niessen at Verabella Spa in Beverly Hills.

Special thanks to Lori Modugno, Patty Sicular, and Jill Cohen Perlman at Iconic Focus for helping me all the way through this book. I love you!

Special thanks to Marimekko Finland, Tarja Rantanen at Andiata, Eila Minkkinen Jewelry, and Anniliina Salmi Knitwear Design. Thank you, Ginni at Wilhelmina Models, Corinne at the Model CoOp,

Marie at Grey Model Agency, Carri at STATE Management, and Catherine at CESD Talent Agency.

Thank you to my supportive friends. You know who you are. And thank you, Kiel Kong, Kari Walden, and Meritta Koivisto for your support. Thank you, Maarit, Rita Tainola at Ilta-Sanomat Finland, Kristina Raitala at *Gloria* magazine, Marita Tabermann-Coccaro, and Yael Gitai for your love, support, and sisterhood. Thank you, Randee St. Nicholas—you are one of the most inspiring women I have ever met. Thank you, Sean Sharifi at RiiFii Design and Stephanie Clinesmith at Clinesmith Design. Thank you, Susan Sykes at Eyes on Main. Thank you to Carre Otis, Karla Welch, and Tatjana Patitz.

And finally, a giant thank-you to my family in Finland: my mother, my sister Irina, and her two beautiful children, Jalmari and Lydia. I love you more than words can say.

CREDITS

Makeup and Creative Direction

Riku Campo
@rikucampobeauty on Instagram

Photography / Beauty and Still Life

Samantha Rapp
www.samantharapp.com

Riku Campo's Assistant and Junior Art Director

Miles Holland

Clothing and Accessories Courtesy of

Afle Bijoux
Jewelry as seen on Tatjana, *Natural Beauty*, 106

Andiata
Blouse as seen on Doreen,
Spring—Daughter and Mother, 118

Clothing as seen on Siobhan, *Hollywood Glamour*, 156

Anniliina Salmi Knitwear Design
Knitwear as seen on Sabine, *Modern Chic*, 200

Ariana Boussard-Reifel
Jewelry as seen on Pat, *Summer in Saint-Tropez*, 132, 134

Chus Bures
Jewelry as seen on Ursula, *Artist*, 218

Jewelry as seen on Teresa, *Modern Grunge*, 92

De Beers
Jewelry as seen on Emme, *Classic Glamour*, 111, 194

Delphine-Charlotte Parmentier
Jewelry as seen on Doreen,
Spring—Daughter and Mother, 124

East Village Hats
Hat as seen on Maarit, *Autumn in New York*, 141

Eila Minkkinen Jewelry
Rings as seen on Sabine, *Modern Chic*, 200

Elena Rudenko
White shirt as seen on Karen,
Spring—Daughter and Mother, 118

Marimekko Finland
Clothing as seen on Tamiyo, *Minimalist*, 98, 100

Mauro Pina
Earrings and necklace as seen on Karen,
Spring—Daughter and Mother, 124

Moises
Feather boa as seen on Siobhan,
Hollywood Glamour, 158

Ricardo Seco
Metallic puffer jacket as seen on Coco, *Colorful*, 172

Solomeina Jewelry
Jewelry as seen on Coco, *Colorful*, 174

THUY Design House
Bomber jacket as seen on Coco, *Colorful*, 172

Vita Kin
Dress as seen on Tatjana, *Natural Beauty*, 106

WeAnnaBe
Blouse as seen on Karen,
Spring—Daughter and Mother, 124

Jacket as seen on Doreen,
Spring—Daughter and Mother, 118

Wedu
Yellow hoodie as seen on Coco, *Colorful*, 172

Xlullan
Dress as seen on Doreen,
Spring—Daughter and Mother, 124

Clothing Stylist

Sabine Feuilloley

Cosmetics and Still Life Stylist

Sarah Guido-Laakso

Eyewear

Eyes on Main in Santa Monica

Makeup

MAKE UP FOR EVER
PROFESSIONAL – PARIS

Hair

Leonor Greyl
PARIS

Hairstylists and Models Seen in Part I

Page 2: Moiz Alladina for Nancy Donahue and Zelda Josephs; Frankie Foye for Lana Ogilvie

Page 3: Frankie Foye for Ling Tan

Page 5: Moiz Alladina for Emme Aronson

Pages 6 and 8: Frankie Foye for Lana Ogilvie

Page 10: Fred Van De Bunt for Shawna Christensen

Page 12: Carmel Bianco for Maarit Glocer

Page 14: Frankie Foye for Lana Ogilvie

Page 17: Moiz Alladina for Celine Kaplan

Page 18: Yukiko Tajima for Karen Bjornson

Page 20: Rebecca Plymate for Cindy Castiglioni

Page 21: Yukiko Tajima for Karen Bjornson

Page 22: Moiz Alladina for Celine Kaplan

Page 27: Yukiko Tajima for Karen Bjornson

Page 28: Frankie Foye for Lana Ogilvie

Page 31: Moiz Alladina for Nancy Donahue

Page 32: Moiz Alladina for Zelda Josephs

Pages 34 and 38: Yukiko Tajima for Karen Bjornson

Page 41: Rebecca Plymate for Cindy Castiglioni

Page 45: Arbana Dollani for Maarit Glocer

Page 46: Fred Van De Bunt for Tamiyo Hasegawa

Page 47: Staci Child for Elizabeth Roxas-Dobrish

Page 50: Moiz Alladina for Allison Walton

Page 52: Fred Van De Bunt for Gunilla Lindblad

Page 54: Paul Fields for Teresa Boyd

Page 55: Yukiko Tajima for Karen Bjornson

Page 56: Moiz Alladina for Allison Walton

Pages 58, 61–63: Fred Van De Bunt for MaryAnn Elizabeth

Page 64: Frankie Payne for Jenny Brunt; styled by Victoria Addcock for *Gloria* magazine (Finland)

Models Seen on Page 86

Shawna Christensen, Ebony Haith, Gunilla Lindblad, Elizabeth Roxas-Dobrish, Fleure Presner, MaryAnn Elizabeth, Cindy Castiglioni, Mimi Fisher, Coco Mitchell, Tziporah Salamon, Lana Ogilvie, and Tamiyo Hasegawa

Hairstylists for Models Seen in Part II

Arbana Dollani for Maarit, Siobhan, and Tziporah

Carmel Bianco for Pat

Frankie Foye for Tatjana and Ursula

Fred Van De Bunt for Tamiyo

Keiko Hamaguchi for Sabine

Moiz Alladina for Celine and Emme

Paul Fields for Teresa

Rebecca Plymate for Karen, Doreen, and Mimi

Staci Child for Coco and Elizabeth

Cover

Models: Eleanor Simon, Maya Haile Samuelsson, and Cathy Fedoruk | Iconic Focus

Makeup: Riku Campo

Stylist: Joe Delate

Hair: John Ruidant

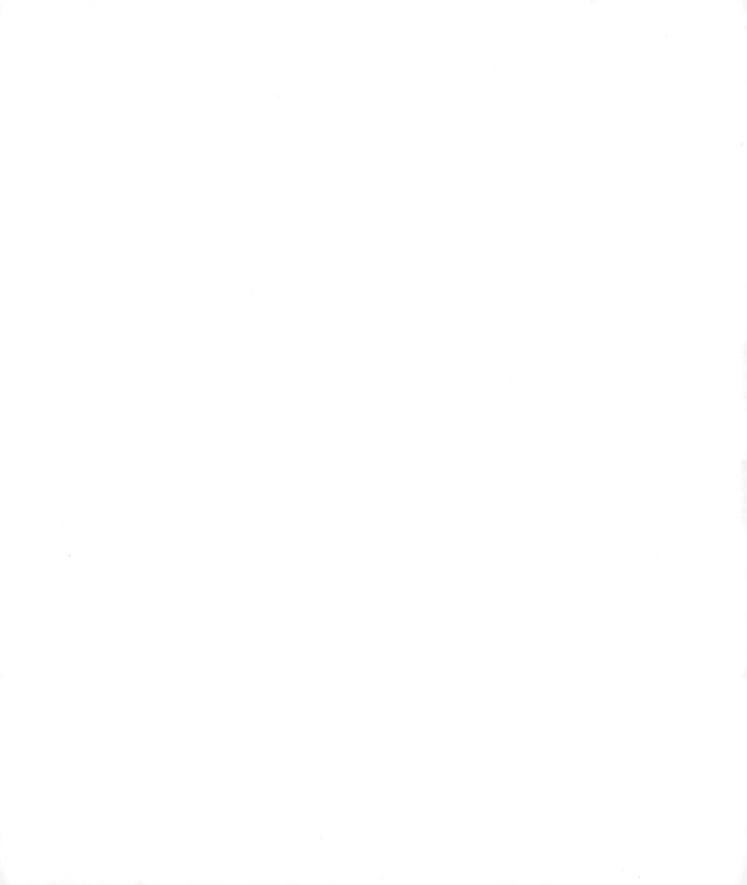